Radiant Passage

Radiant Passage

by
Jeanette H. Fusco

A.R.E. Press • Virginia Beach • Virginia

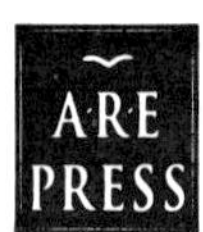

A.R.E. Press
Sixty-Eighth & Atlantic Avenue
P.O. Box 656
Virginia Beach, VA 23451-0656

Library of Congress Cataloging-in-Publication Data
Fusco, Jeanette H., date.
Radiant passage / by Jeanette H. Fusco
p.   cm.
ISBN 0-87604-302-3
1. Fusco, Ray—Health.   2. Abdomen—Cancer—Patients—United States—Biography.   3. Cancer—Alternative treatment.   4. New Age persons—United States—Biography   I. Title.
RC280.A2F874   1993
362. 1'96994347'0092-dc20
[B]   93-6490

The Edgar Cayce psychic readings are identified by a reading number. The original readings are housed at the A.R.E. Library and the Edgar Cayce Foundation in Virginia Beach, Virginia.

Although the sun is setting here,
it's rising where you are.
We have lost you not to the cold dark night,
but to another dawn.

Cynthia Rae Fusco

Acknowledgments

My deepest gratitude goes to my four loving daughters, Cindy, Betsy, Holly, and Gina, who supported and loved me throughout their father's illness; and to Annmarie and Joanne, who steadfastly stood by me during the toughest times, never failing to share their loving kindness. A special thanks goes to Edgar Cayce, whose work has given me so much and without whom I would not have understood our "conscious encounters with spirit." Thanks also to Jon Robertson, my editor, who had infinite patience and fortitude as I brought this book to life.

TABLE OF CONTENTS

INTRODUCTION

My daughter Cindy likened her father's cancer to a runaway freight train. You know how a heavy object set in motion keeps gaining momentum as its own powerful energy takes control? As I thought about it, I had to admit that she was right. The intrusive force roared suddenly into our lives out of the netherworld, first invading and then abducting our entire family. It flung us into an alien place, through weeks of darkness that had only one dimension.

Cancer took us captive in January of 1986 and held us relentlessly until August. We had not given permission to be taken hostage on this terrifying journey. As it unfolded, none of us was permitted to leave, nor did any of us know how it would end. Except for the unusual spiritual experiences that blessed us during this time, we were helplessly lost in a place where we had never walked before.

At the darkest time during his sickness, my husband told us that he wanted others to know about the extraordinary help he had received, even if he didn't escape from the tunnel of illness. Although he had been a logical and analytical engineer throughout his fifty-three years, Ray would have gladly told others how fighting the illness had led him to a conscious awakening in his spiritual life—one that had enabled him to fight his battle on a higher level of awareness.

His strange experiences, which I have come to call "conscious encounters with spirit," pervaded the lives of all of us. They kept us in touch with the heavenly realms during our everyday living, even during the worst of times. These encounters accompanied us through the healing and suffering, the endless waiting, the emotional agony, up until the final passing.

Throughout my life, my mother and I have had many unusual psychic experiences, and the opening to psychic awareness continues to manifest in my daughters. I've always experienced prophetic dreams, and share with my family an ability to communicate telepathically during times of great need. As I grew into adulthood, I sought deeper answers to my frequent questions about life and God and found many of them in the work of the clairvoyant Edgar Cayce. His insights had provided me with a solid background on the subjects of meditation and psychic phenomena. So when Ray began to experience these conscious encounters, it didn't surprise me. What did surprise me, however, was that, after thirty-three years of marriage, he began for the first time to share his inner feelings with me.

Ray's conscious encounters with spirit began as a dramatic out-of-body experience that resulted in tangible proof that there is more to life than we can physically see. Through powerful prayer circles and use of an Oriental healing technique called Reiki, Ray experienced the influence of tremendous energy in his body. In order to find a way to participate actively in his own healing, he learned how to meditate. Then, through Dr. Bernie Siegel's work with exceptional cancer patients, he discovered in himself an uncanny facility with visualization that he was actually able to use to stop his pain, lift his depression, and instill inner peace, even if only for brief intervals.

These encounters continued to confirm for us, not in philosophical concepts but in concrete terms, the rightful part we play in God's plan. Spirit stayed with us throughout this time, helping Ray when he needed it most and helping me through periods that I knew I couldn't have survived alone. Sometimes the assistance seemed like a brick dropping on my head, and at others it was subtle and gentle. I often wondered what form the assistance would take next, but it never disappointed me, even in my darkest hours.

During that time and probably because I needed God so desperately, I can truly say that I accepted these encounters with the feeling and attitude that they were rightfully mine. Even when things seemed their most bleak, I knew with certainty that they would continue.

Ray said that sharing these extraordinary experiences might somehow open the door—if only a crack—for others in need. He would have wanted to support others, whether those who were sick or their family members who loved them so much. Toward the end of his nearly eight months of sickness, he felt it important to reveal the details of these encounters, even though the discoveries he made along the way may seem strange and unorthodox.

Ray left us on August 10 of that year and never had the opportunity to share what he experienced with anyone but his family—myself and our four daughters. It is the purpose of this book to recount it for him from the detailed daily journals I kept during his illness.

These extraordinary spiritual phenomena, along with many others, accompanied us throughout our journey, when the Holy Spirit finally lifted him to the light for his radiant passage into the arms of God. It is all true. Many questions are still with us, but I know if even one individual or one family can find helpful insights in our story, then Ray's terrible suffering was not in vain, but for a noble and loving purpose.

It is difficult for us, even now, to understand the unusual

incidents that surrounded those emotionally intense eight months, although we can't deny the varied ways in which we perceived them at the time. It is my hope and I know Ray's, too, that you take from this story anything that may help you. In doing so, Ray's desire to help others who might be traveling the path that he walked may be fulfilled.

My daughters and I sincerely hope that we, too, can be as brave and courageous as Ray was during his physical war when it comes time for our own transitions. We are greatly comforted, knowing that he was victorious on the spiritual plane, and are deeply grateful that we had been privileged to witness his triumph so intimately.

Jeanette H. Fusco
Ivyland, Pennsylvania
January, 1993

CHAPTER ONE

DIAGNOSIS

(January 1-15)

I chose a white down jacket from the long rack of tightly jammed sale items, held it up in front of me, and looked into the full-length mirror. It's a trivial thing to recall with such clarity, but I still visualize the moment clearly. Over my shoulder I saw my husband Ray watching, and the sudden grimace on his face startled me. Turning around quickly, I asked him what was the matter. We had left the house early that Saturday morning in January, 1986, hoping to reap the benefits from the after-Christmas sales. The crowded department store was brightly lit and the glaring overhead lights magnified his paleness. A pang of fear raced through me. Glancing over at my daughter Betsy, I caught a look of anxiety on her face, too.

"What's wrong?" I repeated softly to Ray.

His brown plaid jacket was unzipped and the protrusion of his stomach was unmistakable. He was heavy, about 190 pounds, but this bulge was different and quite noticeable. Putting his hand on his stomach, he said, "It's just like a rock. Feel this."

I reached over and pressed lightly on his stomach and felt the board-like rigidity. Betsy leaned over and probed gently. She strongly asserted her R.N. training when she told him,

"Dad, I think we'd better get to the hospital and have you checked out. I don't think we should wait."

"What do you think it is?" I asked her.

"He may have a blockage in his intestines," she said.

We bought the white jacket, quickly left the store, and headed for the hospital. Ray had always been in good health. At fifty-three, except for minor knee surgery, he had never experienced serious illness. "I don't have time to be sick," he would always say. In our thirty-three years together, I couldn't even remember him complaining of a headache; sore throats and colds were about it. He had difficulty relating to people who were ill, because he had experienced so little illness himself. Not that he wasn't kind and helpful to them, but he just couldn't understand what it meant to be sick. Our four daughters and I often teased him that he had been saving it for "the big one." He had always been the caretaker, and now I was worried and apprehensive.

Ray insisted on driving to the hospital that morning, and I noticed that his hands were white as he gripped the wheel tightly. I wondered what he was thinking. I glanced quickly at his pale, serious face and wished desperately that he'd say something to me, but his eyes were focused straight ahead. At times of turmoil, he always retreated into himself and couldn't reach out to me. As much as I loved him, this habit of withdrawal had been a great source of frustration to me in all those years of marriage. Whenever he did it, communication would break down, and I'd be left to guess what he was thinking and feeling.

Ray had a dry wit, and many of his friends enjoyed his humor because they never knew whether he was kidding them or not. Sometimes his remark had a two-way cut that hit the mark directly, but often it went over their heads. We had many laughs together over these situations and would crack up occasionally over ridiculous things. Ray was extremely energetic, quite impatient, and did everything in a hurry. Life was an adventure to Ray, and he approached it with enthusiasm. He was usually easygoing, but he had a moody side, too. I learned to use humor a lot, getting him to laugh with me to pull him out of his sporadic dark habit of withdrawing into himself. Then he'd grab me and hug me and burst out laughing despite himself.

Back in September Ray had gone into the short procedure unit to have torn ligaments in his knee repaired. Prior to surgery, a complete medical checkup showed that everything was fine. During the operation, the doctor was surprised to find some old fractures in his knee, but repair was complete and uncomplicated. Ray's recovery was rapid, and it seemed more a nuisance to him than anything else because it slowed him down. Before long however, he was back to his energetic self, expectedly favoring the knee.

October had passed uneventfully. Ray was an electronics engineer and had been doing consulting work during that time which caused him to travel extensively. He had to limit himself to clients that were in his driving area because he still had problems walking around the airport. That autumn, we were living alone for the first time, after many years of rearing children, and we were enjoying the freedom immensely. We were finally able to go out for dinner and a movie or attend local events on the weekend without having to worry about kids at home.

Around Thanksgiving time and his fifty-third birthday, Ray had complained of feeling tired and thought perhaps he had been working too hard. I suggested a checkup, but he refused, reminding me that he had had enough for awhile. "After all," he asked, "didn't I get a clean bill of health after my knee surgery?" I reluctantly agreed.

During the December holidays, our house was chaotic. With people coming and going and daughters and grandchildren dashing in and out, preparations for Christmas were in full swing. Ray continued to work, but he seemed worn out.

He had no blatant, gross symptoms that I could see, although he did mention to me that he was taking laxatives. I was concerned and made a vow that in the next week I would insist that he see the doctor.

Ironically, the Christmas holidays had turned into a nightmare when a virus invaded the household and passed itself around in a chain reaction, downing us like dominoes. Again we assumed that his tiredness and dizziness was from this virus. We did manage to visit my brother and sister-in-law shortly after Christmas, and they both remarked that Ray didn't look good. His dark hair emphasized his paleness, and his skin had a grayish cast. He seemed weary most of the time, and because Ray was normally energetic, his lethargy was pronounced.

His disinterest spilled over into everything, and any physical exertion became an effort for him. All he wanted to do was rest. The sparkle in his big hazel eyes wasn't there any more, and his quick and easy step had diminished almost to a drag. His otherwise mercurial personality was now buried somewhere under a heavy layer of depression, and his tall body seemed to stoop as though under a burden. This all happened so quickly that I didn't know what to think, yet, on the way to the hospital that morning, something nagged at me that this was more than just a virus.

The swerving of the car jerked me abruptly back from my memory delving. Now I focused in on the hospital, which I could see looming upward behind the bypass exit. It stood solemn and brown against the cold, faded-blue January sky of the Philadelphia suburbs where we lived. Apprehension gripped me again. I told myself that it was silly, that nothing was drastically wrong, but the sickly feeling wouldn't leave me. Betsy dropped us off and left to find a babysitter for her four-year-old son, Luke. "I'll be back, Mom," she said. It was Saturday and Luke's nursery school was closed. In the commotion, I had almost forgotten our grandson was with us.

Betsy was our second born, and she had a quiet and reserved demeanor, but this was only what she presented outwardly. Inwardly she was extremely perceptive, caught somewhere between her instinctive awareness and cold, hard logic. Physically she was petite, bordering on delicate, with dark brown hair and huge hazel eyes that missed nothing. When she looked at you, her intensity could make you feel uncomfortable. She was tiny, bright, and rather shy when she was little, but her iron will sustained and balanced her. That January, Betsy was twenty-five years old, divorced, and struggling to raise an eight-year-old daughter and a four-year-old son alone. I was thankful that she was with us that morning.

Ray and I walked into the emergency room and we were fortunate. Miraculously, it wasn't too busy. They immediately brought him back into the examining room, and I waited outside. Without any delay the nurse got him into a hospital gown, and they called me back into the examining room to sit with him. It was so strange for me to see him like that. It had always been one of us on the gurney, with Ray standing by reassuringly.

I quietly waited with him, and disjointed thoughts crept in and out of my mind. The memory of a strange dream from last August started to edge its way into my head. Throughout my life I'd had prophetic dreams. Too many times they'd given me foreknowledge of events that became reality, so since childhood I had learned not to ignore them. My dreams revealed realities to me at many levels, some with deep psychological implications. I remembered how my mother had always been able to predict a death a few weeks or days before the passing of a relative. She would tell me that she saw it in a dream; to my recollection she was always right. She also told me many times that she was the seventh child of a seventh child, and believed in "these things." All four of my daughters have inherited this gift of "second sight" in one form or another.

Back in August, I'd had a terrifying dream, although at the time I could make nothing of it. As I silently waited there that day with Ray, the images of the dream poured vividly through my mind. That summer morning I had awakened, not realizing that it had been a dream. It was so real to me that I was totally disoriented, and its imagery haunted me for days. I pulled it apart from both psychological and spiritual points of view, but I couldn't get a grasp on its meaning. My friends offered many theories and interpretations, but none fit or felt right to me.

In the dream, I had seen Ray pulled under the water by a gigantic snake which transformed itself into an octopus. He had deliberately entered the water, and I tried to save him. I didn't know what it meant then, but it gave me a terrible floating anxiety for a long time afterward. That morning at the hospital, I consciously pushed the dream from my mind, though it took great effort. I wondered why on earth I should suddenly remember it. Mercifully, I wouldn't know what the dream meant until nearly a year later.

I saw the doctor approaching, and my focus shifted back to the large white room. I was acutely aware again of where we were. He remarked how very pale Ray was. He was sure that he was anemic and ordered blood tests immediately. Ray's blood pressure reading was satisfactory; however, the emergency room doctor was concerned with the bloating and rigidity of Ray's stomach. The doctor advised us that he would return as soon as they ran the blood tests. Then he left.

Ray and I talked softly about insignificant things and I held his hand, wondering if he were as frightened as I was. I remembered that Betsy would be back soon. We waited impatiently for the test results. I felt disoriented and out of sync, and I realized how badly I wanted to go home. The overhead lights were too bright, casting a harsh glare on the shiny metal of the instruments and paraphernalia surrounding us. The medicinal smells and the foreign sounds all ran together, and the whole aura of the place was suddenly threatening to me. The panic rose up from my stomach and worked itself into my throat. The setting of the room bounced around me like a new bad dream.

I thought of our other daughters: Cindy, the sensitive visionary of the family, off skiing in the mountains that weekend; Gina, our prophetic dreamer, who was attending a semester of college in England; and Holly, our natural intuitive, at home. Praying that I wouldn't have dreadful news to tell them, I turned and saw the doctor coming toward us again. He reported that the blood work had come back. The red count was down to 8, indicating significant anemia. They discovered that there was intestinal bleeding which was the cause of the anemia. He explained that there was a slow leak into the intestines and, although Ray had not been able to detect it, it must have been going on for an extensive period of time.

We were amazed at what he was saying. Ray told him that he had been fine at the end of October. He couldn't believe that in two months all this could happen without his detection. The anemia explained his dizziness and tiredness of the last few weeks. Ray mentioned to the doctor that he had started feeling tired in December and that it was now only the beginning of January. "How could this happen so quickly?" he asked, shocked and visibly upset.

The doctor then performed a rectal examination on Ray and detected a growth. He thought it must be a blockage, but wanted to consult the surgeon. My stomach turned over and I felt sick. I wanted to say, "You have the wrong person here—he's all right." But somewhere deep inside I knew he really wasn't, and I was so apprehensive of what lay ahead. The surgeon suddenly appeared, introduced himself, and then asked me to leave. A nurse abruptly jerked the curtains around the bed and shut me out. I walked outside to the waiting room and was relieved to see that Betsy was back. We sat and waited together. Wait in the waiting room—that's exactly what you do. It struck me funny at that moment, and the wait seemed forever.

The nurse finally came out and brought us back in. The surgeon had completed his examination and he, too, had felt a large growth in the colon and wanted to look at it more thoroughly through the proctoscope. They admitted Ray for studies and started transfusions, which he assured us would make him feel better.

A proctoscope exam and a lower GI series of x-rays were scheduled for the next morning. Paramount to their concern was the bloating and rigidity of the abdomen, but they would not venture an opinion until the tests were completed. The surgeon was direct, yet I sensed his concern. He was extremely clear and radiated capability and knowledge. There was no coldness or abruptness in his demeanor, so I felt a little more comfortable. However, I had had no dealings with him and I intended to ask my friends who knew him for their opinions. Ray was taken upstairs to the fifth floor, and Betsy and I went into the coffee shop while they got him ready and into bed. We sat in silence. The uncertainty of what was happening seemed to be floating somewhere over my head. Terror was now turning into detached numbness, and I was lost, wandering in the shadows. I had no time even to begin to digest what was happening.

Thoughts of my three other daughters and also Ray's mom tugged at me. Cindy, our eldest, had gone to the mountains for the weekend. How would I reach her? I wasn't sure she had left a telephone number. Holly, our third daughter, could be called at home, and Gina could be reached overseas. We finished our coffee and looked for a telephone.

When Holly answered, I tried not to sound too upset. I knew she would be devastated, and I dreaded telling her. She immediately picked up my anxiety and said she would come right away. Holly was twenty-four years old, married, and had two children. She was tall and slim, with auburn hair, freckles, and green eyes. She was our jokster; very bright, gregarious, and aggressive. Scottish genes from her father's maternal ancestors and Irish genes from mine determined her Gaelic coloring. She was often teased about her Italian last name. Holly resembled me in coloring and freckled skin, whereas my other girls had Ray's dark hair, hazel eyes, and fair skin. We were a real melting pot of a family with my Irish-German heritage and Ray's Scottish, Dutch, and Italian ancestry. Holly was unabashedly verbal and had always been able to communicate more freely with her father than her sisters, expressing herself in an unrestricted way.

She told me that it would take her about an hour to get to the hospital. As for my mother-in-law, Eva, we decided to wait until we left the hospital and had arrived home before calling her. We would wait to call Cindy and Gina, too. The phone contact with Holly grounded me somewhat for a short time, but the barrage of anxiety soon overwhelmed me again. The elevator lifted us up to the fifth floor, and we found Ray's room. The nurses had settled him in, and the first of two transfusions were begun. The afternoon moved in quickly, contradicting my sense of time, and I saw that Ray was exhausted after the extensive examinations and all the chaos.

Betsy and I had been sitting with him for about an hour when Holly arrived. She was nearly frantic, and we tried desperately to calm her down before she went into his room. It was difficult for her to see her father lying in bed so ill. I related strongly to how she felt. She composed herself quickly, and he was happy to see her. We all sat and talked for awhile, but no one mentioned the word cancer. Then we realized that Ray was exhausted, so we decided to go home and come back after dinner. Drowsiness took him before we left the room. Holly came home with us while her husband took care of their two little girls. She wanted to be with us.

Once home, I placed the first of many calls, locating Gina in

Northern Ireland at her fiance's home. She was terribly shaken, as I was relaying it. She wanted to take the first plane home.

Gina was the youngest of her sisters and always overflowed with emotions. She was twenty years old and reacted passionately to most situations. She had inherited an exotic intensity from the Italian side of Ray's family. Slender, average in height with long brown hair, she had big, light hazel eyes fringed with long dark lashes like her father. She was emotionally and psychically sensitive and intense in her attitudes. Because she was the baby of the family, we would sometimes forget that she was no longer a child. I thought to myself that I would have given anything to spare her this worry. However, I knew that she would be all right when the initial storm of information had been digested. After she settled down, she agreed with me that we really didn't know anything certain yet, and it would be better to wait.

Cindy had not left me a phone number. The only information that I remembered was that she would be staying at a friend's cabin outside a big ski town. I realized I didn't have the name of her friend, but I did recall the name of the ski resort. I decided to call the police in the resort town to see if they had any suggestions. They advised me to call the ski lodge in the area where everyone eventually showed up. The lodge office personnel promised to put a note on the bulletin board at the bottom of the lift, but it was already late afternoon and Cindy had probably left. It was a chance anyway, so I asked them to go ahead and post the note. There were also non-physical ways in which I could reach Cindy, and later, when I was alone, I would try.

My mother-in-law, Eva, was silent when I told her about Ray. She had health problems herself, and sometimes it took her a few minutes to comprehend what was being said. After I told her, however, she tried to sound optimistic, although it seemed like denial to me. "He'll come through just fine. He'll be all right," she said, trying to assure us. I wished I could agree with her, and at that moment I was trying hard. We left Eva's and headed home.

It was almost supper time when we realized that we hadn't eaten much all day. Although no one had an appetite, I decided to fix dinner anyway. It gave me something to do. There was only trivial conversation and soft weeping around the table during the meal. We all fumbled under the enormous weight of something terrible descending upon us. None of us were able to comprehend or express our feelings about the day.

Ray called us later before we had a chance to leave for the hospital and told us he was worn out and would rather get a good night's sleep. I felt some relief because I needed time to digest the day's events. Although I wanted to be with him, exhaustion triumphed, and I was thankful to sit down and rest. Frustrated by my inability to contact Cindy by phone, I was determined to communicate with her in another way. Many times our family had shared telepathic communication or received strong messages in dreams, when one of us was in trouble.

A few years before, Holly had had a terrible car accident. I remembered how Betsy, then twenty, came into our room at 3:00 in the morning to wake me up. She told me that Holly was in serious trouble. Well, of course, what mother wouldn't worry? But it wasn't until 5 a.m. that we learned that Holly had been taken to the hospital with serious head injuries sustained in a car accident. From the smashed clock on the dashboard, we knew that the crash had occurred at exactly 3 a.m.—the precise time Betsy awakened me.

When the children were small, Ray traveled a great deal in his job, mostly via commercial airlines. I remember once when he was flying in from Washington, D.C., and the children and I were at home waiting for him. I heard the garage door lift and told the children, "Here comes Daddy. Go down and open the den door." They ran down to open the door but came back upstairs to tell me there was no one there. Then, I knew he was in some sort of danger from the wave of anxiety that swept over me. Shortly afterward Ray called to tell me that the plane had run into trouble, but landed safely. They had hit severe downdrafts while flying, and a number of passengers were thrown around the plane and injured. He didn't want me to hear about it on the news.

We have experienced many similar events together and acknowledged the extent of our mental and spiritual network. I was able to reach all my girls and Ray, too, at times, using telepathy or, as I called it, "mind conveyance." They would contact me or I them, after the psychic connection had been made. That night, I decided to try to reach Cindy telepathically, praying that I would find her and that she'd telephone me.

Years before, I had been introduced to the work of a psychic named Edgar Cayce, who had given thousands of readings until his death in 1945. Called the "sleeping prophet" even today, he included in his work the practice of meditation, with which I later became acquainted. In many ways, meditation helped me keep an even keel in my emotional life. It calmed me when I was stressed and, because I was prone to be somewhat overly energetic, it dissipated some of that abundance of energy. I would focus on colors during meditation, associating them with the different spiritual energy centers or chakra points in my body, and I would emerge refreshed. Meditation always quieted my mind and got me to a place of inner quiet and peace. That night, however, deep meditation proved to be difficult to achieve because my mind was racing like a whirlwind. Still, in order to "find" Cindy, I tried to grow calm.

Settling myself down, I began to relax into meditation. I visualized rays of the color violet and sent my thoughts riding on them to Cindy. The image of my twenty-nine-year-old elder daughter came clearly to my mind's eye and entered my inner focus. I saw her short, dark, shiny hair and intense hazel eyes with a speck of dark brown in one clear iris. Suddenly, I felt her keenly. Cindy was the smallest, physically, of her sisters, dry of wit, perceptive, and intelligent. Nothing got by her. Her features were small and perfect. She greatly resembled my gentle Irish grandmother, Sarah Ann. Her personality was mercurial; her natural sensitivity and intuitiveness were often apparent, and she used these two assets like antennae. A humanitarian, she showed great empathy for others. At the time, Cindy had been working in the space program as a chemist, supervising a materials development lab, but her goal was to become a physician.

To use telepathy, I had learned that holding a picture in my hand enhanced the contact. I called to her silently within myself, praying that she would hear me and respond. If Ray had to undergo any kind of emergency surgery, Cindy would be shattered if she were not here. After my best try, hours passed; still no phone call. We went to bed, then, and I prayed that Cindy had heard me.

In the morning, Holly, Betsy, and I returned to the hospital. Even though it was Sunday, the surgeon had called the radiologist in to do a lower GI series. After we arrived, Ray was brought up to the fifth floor examining room where the surgeon did the proctoscope exam and immediately sent a small sample biopsy to the lab. Not long after, Ray was returned to his room. The surgeon came in then and abruptly stated, "There is a large growth in the colon. From what I see, 99 chances out of 100 are that it's malignant. I feel it's pretty well confined to that area, but I want to wait for the GI tests to confirm this, to see if it's completely blocking the colon."

As we listened wide-eyed, he went on to say that if it were a complete blockage, he'd operate immediately, remove the growth, and put a colostomy bag on for thirty to sixty days until the colon healed. Then he'd go in and reconnect the colon. I remembered how coldly objective he was. At the time,

I felt as if he were talking about removing a hangnail; but there was more. "If the blockage is not complete," he declared, "we'll operate, remove the growth with some colon on either side, suture the colon together, and that will be that."

And that will be that? How short and simple and final the proclamation had sounded. And that will be that. I wasn't able to get the sentence out of my mind for a long time. Evidently he noticed my stunned reaction to his report and tried to assure us that the latter was pretty routine, that he had done many of them. He told us that he had also thought of scheduling a CAT scan to explore for additional tumors.

The results of the GI tests finally came back; they showed no other masses. The CAT scan idea was scrapped. The surgeon was pleased with Ray's overall good physical condition and said that this, along with his age, would work to his advantage. The GI tests also showed that the blockage was not total, so they would proceed with the removal of the tumor plus some of the colon on either side. We felt a little relieved to learn this.

The surgeon outlined the "game plan." I knew I would have to get used to these metaphors; I was annoyed that Ray's surgery was being compared to what I was beginning to perceive as a football game. "Preparation for this type of surgery will consist of seventy-two hours of cleansing the colon," the surgeon announced. "Surgery will be scheduled for Wednesday morning." I knew that they had not decided exactly what was causing the bloating and rigidity, and would only know after surgery. There were a number of doctors involved, besides the surgical team. The oncologist (cancer specialist) and our family physicians, who were internists, joined them.

Then we heard the confirmation from the lab. It was definitely cancer. Even though we had been warned from the start that it most likely would be, hearing the positive confirmation rolled over us like a wave of terror. We were emotionally knocked down and wiped out. We would later learn that this form of cancer was rare and very aggressive. We tried so hard to regroup and show strength in the hope that it could be completely removed.

The doctors were amazed that the tumor had reared its ugly head in so short a time with no overt symptoms. Ray had taken a positive, optimistic attitude and wanted to get past the surgery. I felt my emotional self trying to hide, leaving my physical self to assimilate this awful diagnosis. I felt as if I were watching the scene from another place, as an outside observer. The unreality was constant, overwhelming, and frightening.

That afternoon, Cindy walked into Ray's room with her close friend Cathy. I was elated and relieved to see them. Deep concern was on Cathy's face and Cindy was solemn and quiet. I knew that she was especially shaken. She told me that she had felt my devastation the night before at about 11:30 p.m.—the exact time I was "calling" to her in my meditation. They both told me that Cindy was up half the night telling Cathy that something was wrong. But there had been no telephones to use. She had spent a sleepless night knowing that I was calling to her and that something was very wrong.

She had left the lodge early the day before, so she missed the message on the bulletin board. She only saw it when she went down to the ski lodge early the next morning to telephone me. I wasn't home, so she called Grandma Eva, who was so mixed up that Cindy couldn't make sense of anything she said, except that her father was gravely ill. She called Holly's husband and he filled her in. That's when she returned home. Cindy is psychically supersensitive, and I realized that I shouldn't have worried about her not hearing me "call" her.

I reached Gina again and informed her of the impending necessary surgery that Wednesday. We decided to wait for the outcome of the surgery, then I would call her at school in

England. In the meantime, Holly and her little girls, Rachael and Lindsay, stayed with me at home all week and gave me much needed support.

Ray was quite uncomfortable for the next few days from the preparations for his surgery, but otherwise he was feeling better overall. The transfusions gave him a great boost as promised. We all spent that Tuesday visiting with him and trying to keep his mind occupied as much as possible. Ray professed positiveness when we saw him that evening and it anchored us somewhat, but I was suspicious, especially when he wouldn't make eye contact with me.

The next day was surgery. Before we left him, I sensed his edginess. I knew how worried he would have been if he had permitted himself to acknowledge the harsh truth. He had great difficulty in communicating sensitive issues, and I had to leave him alone. I didn't want to try to lead him into any conversations that he didn't want. There had always been an unbridgeable chasm between us because of his inability to express himself. Many times I felt his anguish because he could not speak about something but was powerless to help. It wasn't the words that he couldn't put together; it was the emotional content that went with the words.

Most often throughout our thirty-three years of marriage, I had to be the one who initiated a sensitive discussion. Sometimes it would work, but most of the time it would make him angry. Often I was forced to speak, whether he answered me or not. At least I knew that he always heard me. I pulled away from my thoughts and heard Ray as he started to tell me about the medical preparation for that night and the following day. His engineering training made him very methodical and time-oriented; knowing the schedule let him realize what to expect. I knew this somehow helped him. When it was time for us to leave, he looked deeply into my eyes, and I felt a separation between us begin. I didn't want to leave him alone. All we could do was tell him how much we loved him and that we'd be back before the scheduled 9 a.m. surgery.

After we got home, he called to tell me that he had managed to calm himself. His face came into my mind's eye. I saw his dark hair against his pale, worried face, the intensity of his hazel eyes, and a lump closed my throat. I could not speak, and I needed a moment to gather myself. He just wanted to get it over with; I wished it were finished, too. I cried out to my loving God that night to help Ray, and I asked for a positive outcome to the surgery. I was exhausted and sleep came immediately.

The phone was ringing from some faraway place, and I couldn't wake up. Totally disoriented, I felt the phone in my hand and heard myself saying hello. The clock said 7 a.m., and Ray was telling me, "They're coming for me at 7:15. I'm the first one scheduled for surgery." His voice was starting to sift through my grogginess. I was acutely annoyed that they had changed the time. Now I was wide awake. We talked for a few minutes, and he related that the operation should take about two hours. It would be foolish for us to sit in the hospital that long, and I couldn't possibly get over there in fifteen minutes to see him before he went in. "I've got to go," he said. "They're here for me."

I told him I loved him and that we were all praying for him. We would be sending him light, and we'd be there when it was over.

I was soon out of bed dialing Cindy and, after passing the news to her, I called Betsy who was already at her job in another local hospital. "I'll wait for your call when it's over, Mom," she told me. Cindy, Holly, my close friend Joanne, and I decided to meet for breakfast at the diner near the hospital. Joanne joined us to lend moral support. I appreciated her company because she was steadfast, sensitive, and she knew about cancer from caring for her mother. Joanne had been my longtime friend and my partner in my many metaphysical studies. We felt spiritually attuned to each other.

In the waiting room that morning, we all felt that sitting down was hopeless; so we paced and spoke of things that had little meaning. At last, we were notified that Ray was out of surgery and that the surgeon would be with us shortly. We all stood up, anxiously anticipating the doctor's appearance.

He came in almost immediately, looking disheveled and overtired. I noticed that his face mask was askew, hanging halfway off his neck and down onto his chest. Visibly upset, he sat down. His face was pale and solemn. "The news is not good," he said. "It did not go well. There are massive tumors attached to the peritoneum, and it's extensive and inoperable. I've removed a very large mass in the lower abdomen to reduce the bulk and make Ray more comfortable. The initial growth is on the outside of the colon, but it has perforated through the colon and spread into and throughout the abdominal cavity."

He went on to tell us that this particular cancer secretes a fluid that carries and spreads the cancer cells. It was this fluid that had caused the bloating and rigidity. He told us that he had taken out the largest mass, but that it was only about 20 percent of what was in there. The growths were attached to the walls of the abdomen. To extract them would be life threatening because tissue would have to be removed with each growth and this could not be done safely. Some were the size of golf balls, he said. During the operation he had consulted with the oncologist about removing the colon. They both decided it would be life threatening and would serve no purpose because the growths were not in the colon. He said he couldn't believe that the cancer hadn't yet invaded any other major organ.

I looked around, wondering to whom he was talking. I didn't see anyone else in the room but us, and I was confused. This was a gross mistake. He couldn't be saying these things to me. A soundproof barrier went up in my mind, and I would not listen. The doctor was a blur of green. His mouth was moving, but nothing was being converted in my head. All I saw was a green shirt and pants; my focus was on the white mask hanging crookedly down onto his chest. I wondered if he knew his mask was hanging that way.

Then I looked around the room to see where I was. I noticed that Cindy, Holly, and Joanne were in my nightmare, too. I thought how odd it was that we were all together in this dream. Maybe if one of us would move, we could all wake up. Joanne was silent in the corner. I saw her shaking her head, but the movement was too slow and had a dreamlike quality. I still couldn't wake up and stop the nightmare. I crashed back into reality and heard the doctor asking, "Do you want to know anything?"

We were all struck dumb and just sat looking at one another vacantly, not seeing or comprehending anything. The surgeon rambled on that he had left a tube in the abdomen for drug therapy because the oncologist had suggested this, and on and on. He advised us that he had not spoken to Ray about any of this yet. Numbly I turned away, unable to take in anything he was saying. I was cold and could not feel my body; I was floating off somewhere. If only I could have removed myself from this alien place. The desire to run almost conquered me. But I held tightly to my chair to anchor myself so I wouldn't get up, race out of the room, and run screaming down the hall. Please God, I heard myself asking, come down and take me away from this insanity. I wanted to see Ray. I heard someone asking where he was, and I realized it was I.

The surgeon told me he was still in the recovery room but would be down shortly. "Miraculously," he said, "he came through the surgery very well. You'll see him coming by the door in just a little while on his way back to his room."

Cindy and Holly asked some questions, but I was past understanding anything. I only recognized their voices.

"I must get back to the O.R. I've got more surgery sched-uled," the surgeon announced and started moving toward the door. Turning around, he told us to talk with the oncologist, who was the drug specialist. He had made an appointment for us with him for the following morning. The surgeon had completed his part. Dr. Thomas, the oncologist, would be handling Ray's case from then on. We automatically thanked him, and I watched his back moving out through the doorway as he disappeared.

No one moved or said a word because we could not believe what we had just heard. How could this be? Ray had been fine six weeks ago. What happened? I heard Holly crying softly, "Not my Dad."

Cindy was in shock and just sat there, her face blank. Joanne and the girls moved over to me, and we all huddled together. I realized that I was sobbing. The actuality was unacceptable. It was hanging in the air, and I would not let it in. I was sure they must have made a mistake. Cindy was stunned. The tears rolled down her face as she softly wept. Holly kept moaning insistently, "Not my Dad."

Joanne tearfully tried to comfort us all. I felt it would have been better if Ray and I had both been killed in an accident than this; I could not bear it. One by one they repeated to me what the doctor had just said: There were no predictions that he could make; the prognosis was not good because of the extent of the growths, but in Ray's favor were his age and his otherwise good health. The surgeon said that he had seen too many unpredictable outcomes to even venture a guess what would happen. However, I could not be consoled.

Someone remembered that Betsy had to be called at work. Cindy came back and told us, "Betsy will be with us as soon as she can get here."

"We have to call Gina, too," I whispered, thinking how awful it was going to be. The nightmare continued, and I could not accept any part of it. I kept waiting to wake up. I was so sure it was a terrible dream. I felt as if I were walking a sharp edge between dreaming and reality. What and how would I tell Ray? My concern for him was overwhelming. Joanne had to leave, and I hugged her and thanked her for being there.

We heard a gurney rolling down the hall. It was Ray's. We rushed out into the corridor to make sure that it was he. I suddenly realized that part of my fear was that I might not see him again after what we had just heard. He was alert and looked surprisingly good. That settled us all down. His presence quieted and calmed us because he was with us. "I just saw Joanne and talked to her a bit," he said. We couldn't believe how well he looked and how awake he was after such extensive surgery. Then he asked me if I had spoken to the doctor and what he had said. My response was spontaneous and partial. "They found more tumors than they expected, but they're going to treat them with drugs. The surgeon took a large tumor out and left a tube in your stomach to use for chemotherapy," I told him.

He nodded and said, "Oh. O.K."

How much he fully comprehended was impossible to know, but I didn't volunteer any more information then. With this, he dozed off. We were amazed and couldn't get over how good he looked. I stared at his peaceful face and found that what we had been told was too incredible to accept. Maybe it was all in my mind. Perhaps the doctor had the wrong person; I would double-check. They wheeled him down to his room, and we retreated to the solarium to regroup, stare at each other, and fall back into the void.

I really knew what the doctor had said, but the words and the emotions they conveyed were like an outside tangible shape, alive yet synthetic, that would not mesh into my thought processes. I started to project into the future. My heart hurt so badly that I felt it travel up and weep out through my eyes. We talked some more, but I couldn't keep my concentration focused. Everyone had to constantly repeat words to me.

Betsy came rushing into the waiting room in her nurse's whites, completely shaken and sobbing. We hugged her into our circle, and the girls shared with her what the doctor had said. I knew that it was even more difficult for her, because she saw the reality of sickness in her nursing. She listened to her sisters all speaking at once, then quickly left and hurried down the hall to see her father. I followed her rigid, solemn figure to his room. Her face brightened when she saw how good he looked. She checked the I.V. and everything else until she was satisfied that all was in order. We sat with him awhile longer, then it was time to leave the hospital for a short time; they wanted him to sleep.

We walked down the sterile white corridor, silent, separate, each in her own thoughts. Someone pressed the elevator button, and we found ourselves in the main lobby. The automatic doors swung open, passing us through to the cold winter air of the outside world. We were amazed that nothing had changed. I looked around at the drab brown lawn and the overcast sky. The sun was partially out, pale on that bleak January day in 1986, mirroring our feelings. I felt strangely disconnected to the everyday movement around me—the hubbub and noise in the parking lot. It was blurred, like pictures with no sound. It pushed through my ears as buzzing and echolalic, and at first I could not decipher it. No one had anything to say because we knew that what lay ahead would be even more difficult. We had to stop at Ray's mother's house.

I had prepared her somewhat, but this was no gentle thing— it was monstrous and I hoped I could tell her calmly. Ray had been her baby, her child and son for fifty-three years. I could not anticipate nor comprehend how she would feel. She greeted us at the door as we arrived en masse. Her frailty seemed more pronounced, and I hoped that I could speak. Cindy pulled the blinds up to let more light in. Maybe this would help, or did it really matter? It gave Cindy something to do. I related to her first the positive things and skipped over other information. I could not tell her just yet all the frightening things the doctor had said.

Silence. All she said was "Umm hmm." More silence, while we waited for the information to register.

Finally she said, "You know those coveralls Ray was trying to find for Johnny? Well, Jamesway has them."

She was referring to a Christmas gift Ray could not find for his brother! For a moment I was stunned, until I realized what she was doing. She could not or would not accept the awfulness of what I had just told her. Her mind was rejecting it.

Holly was terribly upset, as she hadn't immediately realized what her grandmother was doing. "Grandma, do you understand how serious this is?"

"Yes, but what can we do?" she sighed.

Our visit was short. Gina still had to be called. Her absence from us left the pang of a large void. Without her presence our circle was broken, and everyone felt it desperately. We were greatly worried about her, for each one of us knew how we would have felt if we had been so far away. When I finally reached Gina, her fiance, Brian, who was involved in his family's large restaurant complex, had come down from Northern Ireland and was now there with her in England. Gina had already called the airport to check flights and had been able to get on a late afternoon plane. She had had an uncertain feeling about Ray's surgery and sensed she would have to leave as soon as possible. I thanked God for the time difference which gave her the space to make the flight and that Brian had been there to help her.

I pictured the vast ocean between us, and it made me cry. Gina told me she had already called her college here and would be able to get back in this semester and commute from home. She was a junior now, and it was important that she be able to graduate in May of 1987. Also, I wanted her here with us.

That evening, we sat in the den, dazed, silent, and detached. This alien thing had invaded us, nesting in our midst and distorting our reality. It was something no one could comprehend, much less accept. Cindy was totally shaken and started to babble nervously. Betsy was silent and retreated into herself. Holly was angry and lashed out physically at objects and the general space around her. I just sat and shifted into neutral. I wanted to stay in that middle ground of nonacceptance, non-partaker in reality. At times I was successful, but then I was afraid that I wouldn't come back out.

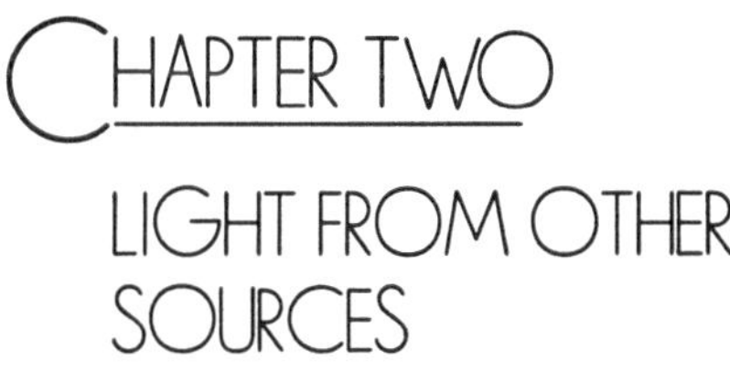

(January 16-20)

The shock of Ray's diagnosis led me into a storm of soul-searching. I never thought a challenge like this would be a part of my life or Ray's. Cancer was for other people, not us. I asked over and over in my mind why this should happen to Ray, and out of my searching emerged a startling question: "Why is Ray taking this path?"

I suddenly felt strongly that somehow, at the soul level, Ray may have been unconsciously using this illness for a deeper purpose. I knew from my study of Edgar Cayce's psychic readings that, "Spirit is the life; mind is the builder; physical is the result." This means that through our own thoughts and actions we create the circumstances of our present or future lives. I believed that, in Ray's case, this was a complex issue, involving many things which included his genetics, karma, and the way he had been trying to solve numerous problems at once. I didn't think his conscious mind had led him to this illness. Who would consciously choose to bring something like this upon himself or herself?

I pondered these questions continually, knowing full well that I was not meant to know the answers—at least not then. I knew that when I entered the other side of dawn, everything would be revealed to me, but for the present I would have to accept his soul's decision, no matter how difficult it was. The depth of my understanding into the nature of the soul and the hidden meaning of life had at least taken me that far.

Throughout childhood, I had an unusual sense of what was going on inside others, but their contradictory outer image always confused me. As I matured, my dreams gave me glimpses into the future or insights into people and coming events. I didn't know where the whisperings originated. Sometimes I listened, other times I ignored them. After I was married, I used to write some of them down on paper, with dates and times. When they came true, even Ray would be amazed, though I never knew whether he believed they were anything more than just coincidence.

It was also at times like those that I had wished he would have been able to communicate what he was feeling. I'd sensed for years that Ray had inner feelings about paranormal events and that he received a great deal of information from his inner self. He would read metaphysical books that I gave him, but his engineer's demeanor was always more comfortable with logic and facts. Yet sometimes, when we were at social gatherings, I would see him across a room, call him silently, and he would quickly turn his beautiful eyes to meet my gaze. I supposed he really didn't know what to do with information that might have come from inside himself. And, like everything else, he never communicated them. Ray was always an interested observer, standing just out of reach and seldom expressing thoughts that were not based on fact. All I knew at that time was that I was hungering for more knowledge, more revelations about God and the universe.

When we moved to Florida in 1964 because of Ray's job in the aerospace industry, I wasn't aware of any groups studying psychic phenomena. Of course, I assumed that there were individuals around who had the kind of spiritual knowledge that I was searching for, but I had no idea where to find them.

I remember visiting a psychic during that time. She told me that my husband would have a serious illness later in life and that I was to remember that it was his soul's choice. If I could accept that premise, it would help me immensely in living through that time. She either could not or would not tell me more. I never gave it another thought, until now.

Around 1968, I happened upon a book, *Many Mansions* (William Morrow, New York, 1968), by Gina Cerminara, about the psychic readings of Edgar Cayce. I was fascinated by the fact that Cayce had been able to relay a vast range of information while in trance. I had never read anything like it. That one little book had filled an inner void with reasonable explanations to my many questions. I could see immediately that Cayce's readings picked up where my church's doctrines left off. The information contained in them told me what I needed to know about the workings of the mind, the cyclic nature of the soul, reincarnation, and how everything fits together. It confirmed what I had sensed inwardly all along and rang so true that I wished I could shout it to the world. The readings contained answers that, until then, I had been taught were nonexistent. They provided explanations for the inequalities of birth, early deaths, sicknesses, and much more.

Cayce left over 14,000 documented stenographic records of the clairvoyant statements he had given for thousands of people over a period of forty-three years. These documents, referred to as "readings," covered the entire range of human thought and are housed at the Association for Research and Enlightenment (A.R.E.) headquarters in Virginia Beach, Virginia. The entire collection is on file for anyone to use, and they are regularly consulted by researchers, doctors, students, writers, investigators, and psychologists.

Many of Cayce's amazing readings concerned health problems, along with various, often unorthodox healing techniques and remedies. I was fascinated to learn about the many spiritual readings he gave on all sorts of subjects. The more I read, the more I wanted to read. Visitors from all over the world still go to the A.R.E. to research, study, and gain knowledge from the readings for the purposes of education and spiritual growth. After *Many Mansions* opened my eyes to Cayce's work, I continued with the definitive biography of his life, *There Is a River*, by Thomas Surgrue, and other books about the contents of the readings.

I immediately took into my heart what I felt was one of the most important principles that Cayce revealed. He said that the sources of illness and all karma "are the meeting of one's own self." Ultimately, we are each responsible for self. I thought about how profound that simple statement is and what truth it contains. It showed me that I am responsible in my life and have to answer for myself. I felt that the word "self" is interchangeable with soul. I saw the word "responsible" in the context of our free will to choose. The principle can be extended to the rearing of our children, where we parents are asked to guide, love, and care for their emotional and physical needs and to prepare them to be responsible for themselves. The principle also extends to our judgment of others when we are unaware of their path in life. We eventually meet our inner selves in health as well as in sickness.

I was also moved by Cayce's readings on the evolution of the soul and how best to pursue our long journey back to God. The soul holds all our positive and negative adventures in unconscious memory, so our good and bad experiences are carried forth into each new life. Positive action helps us evolve toward Christ, whereas negative action, or karma, has to be balanced.

In 1972 we moved back to Pennsylvania where I still reside. During the early seventies and after I had become more familiar with Edgar Cayce's work, people began to pop in and out of my life who were well acquainted with the readings. I've thought about it several times since and wonder how I was drawn to these particular people. I believe that coincidence is

God's anonymity; maybe synchronicity played a part, too. In either case, I welcomed these helpers into my life.

It wasn't long before I joined an A.R.E.-sponsored study group called a Search for God. I loved it. The group, which I joined in 1974, discussed various questions about life, death, and the nature of the soul. It was at that time that I was introduced to the practice of meditation. I was finally among people with whom I could align my beliefs. Unfortunately, after a year, the leader who organized the group moved from the area and the group disbanded. But I continued with the meditation techniques I had learned there. At that time I couldn't find another local study group, so from the Cayce material I moved on, reading all the Jane Roberts' "Seth" books and other writers, such as Brad Steiger, Louise Hay, Holger Kalweit, Elisabeth Kübler-Ross, Richard Bach, Meredith Young, Ram Dass, and Brugh Joy. Suddenly there was an abundance of informational books available on metaphysical topics.

In 1983, I saw a small notice in the local newspaper advertising the forming of a study group leading to understanding and using your psychic ability. It was located in my immediate area. I joined the group and met Annmarie, a very stable and psychically oriented young woman with a great deal of knowledge and experience. Annmarie was teaching a well-grounded series of classes on parapsychology that in large part had been patterned on Cayce's work. Her husband, John, who was also a student of the Cayce material, had been working with alternative healing techniques and visualization programs. Both were certified hypnotists.

When I joined her psychic understanding class, many things began to come into perspective for me. My thinking was still connected somewhat to my Catholic upbringing, and I didn't yet possess the freedom of mind to see that psychic events emanate from our own natural abilities, from the light, and from God. I hadn't fully realized that everyone has this awareness and that it can be developed. Despite my early dream activity, I was initially afraid of developing my psychic ability. I had never had a problem opening my mind to God, but I hadn't understood that our abilities to connect with Him intuitively are also spiritual.

Working with my dreams had been a continuing study for me. I found it fascinating. I approached interpretation mainly from the psychological view then, but now I was able to see how spiritual imagery was another aspect of many dreams. I learned to direct and comprehend the inner messages that I was now allowing to filter through, once I had lost my fear of them, and began to understand how they related to my present physical existence. I started to find the satisfaction and meaning that I had been seeking at that time in my life, to understand my place in the universe and my true relationship with every other soul. I looked at others in this new light of understanding and was able to be more tolerant of their short-comings as well as my own. Although I hadn't believed myself judgmental, I found that I needed some work on that aspect as well. But now I was able to see things differently, because I had a new perspective and new awareness.

Together with other seekers who were searching for spiritual understanding, we explored further psychic events in our lives through the different approaches taught to us. Being with the group seemed to magnify our individual energy. Together we generated and enhanced our abilities in seeking answers as a unit. Annmarie continues to be a dear friend, although she no longer teaches, and so does Joanne, whom I met in Annmarie's group.

I remember how my barriers were lowered during that class in 1983, three years before Ray got sick. It was a good time of life for both of us, and Ray especially enjoyed one particular paranormal experience that resulted from my studies. I had begun receiving answers in my meditations. In the beginning, I obtained so much information that I was skeptical and couldn't accept all that was coming to me. I recall how I asked my higher self to give me tangible proof that my mind wasn't just playing tricks on me. (In metaphysical studies, you should always be skeptical and ask God for validation.) A short time later my answer came, perhaps in an unexpected way, but it was a validation nonetheless.

During meditation, or perhaps it was that relaxed first stage between wakefulness and sleep, I found myself watching what was similar to a moving picture screen with a corner torn down so I could peek over into the contents. I was at a large racetrack. A gorgeous mustard tan horse was in the winner's circle. He was very large and his glossy tan coat glistened in the brilliant sunshine. The colors I saw around me were vivid and distinct; the grass was a bright green, the sky a beautiful blue. In the distance, behind the winner's circle, I could see many colored flags flying atop the stadium in a well-ordered row, waving and cracking sharply in the wind.

Everything was focused precisely; crisp, colorful, and vivid. Lucidly I could see the jockey's brilliant silks as he sat upon this magnificent horse in the middle of the winner's circle. They were putting a horseshoe of bright, multi-colored flowers around his neck. I thought to myself, as I watched this so clearly, how gleaming and healthy this horse's lovely tan coat was. I knew I could pick him out of a thousand horses because of his distinctive coloring. I also knew that his name was *Tanner*. They had named him for his gorgeous, unusual tan shade. I watched for awhile longer, then the scene faded, and I opened my eyes.

It was beyond my understanding why I had seen anything like this because I knew absolutely nothing about racehorses and had no interest in them. I wrote it down anyway, told my family and class about it, and then got the idea to ask Ray to pick up a racing sheet the next day. Maybe we could find the horse's name on it. He didn't take me seriously, even though he said my story was interesting.

I remember it was almost Palm Sunday. The whole horse episode had faded, and we were all together that weekend, just hanging out. Holly was sitting on the floor reading the newspaper, when suddenly she jumped up and yelled, "Mom, your horse won!"

Holly was our family jokster, so I thought she was kidding me. I replied, "Yeah, sure, Holly."

"I'm not kidding, Mom," she said, waving the newspaper at me. "Look here," and she excitedly read me the headline: "Tanner in Upset Victory at Brandywine."

This was in headlines in the sports section; no little one-liner on the back page! How was this to be explained? I had asked for a solid, real confirmation that I could trust my psychic impressions, and I certainly had received solid information, odd though it was. Was this evidence enough to move forward and accept other insights and happenings? I wondered how someone who denies everything but the physical would explain this, but Ray only shrugged his shoulders in confusion. I cut the article out and kept it to remind myself of my solid proof whenever doubt crept in.

Later, Ray said, "Try it again. Maybe you can pick some other horses!" But I knew that this wasn't a matter of picking horses, that this sign had not been given to me for that purpose. Numerous other events occurred during that first year, some as exciting in other ways as the episode just recounted.

Sometime later, I had an extremely vivid dream which I recorded. These occasional dreams had a quality of reality so strong that it set them apart distinctly from what I call "ordinary dreams."

The dream took place in France. I knew it was France from the clothes, hair styles, and decor of the room where I was. The setting was in a bedroom with a large, dark, wooden four-poster bed. Heavy curtains were draped around it. I was dressed in a beautiful golden gown, and my hair, which was dark in the dream, was piled high on my head. I wasn't sure if it was a wig or if my own hair had been done in many ringlets. It was very colorful and real, and Ray was with me.

He was wearing a white shirt made of silk with loose flowing sleeves, dark pants, and high leather boots. It seemed that we were of a higher class, possibly aristocrats, by the mode of dress and the furnishings. We were young and had not been married long. Ray did not look exactly as he does now and neither did I, but I knew it was he. The dream seemed to reflect a setting, a mood, rather than action. I was feeling angry and resentful over some difficulty with intimate communications between us—or rather the lack of it. I couldn't remember the conversation that had brought about my anger, but I wrote the dream down without mentioning it to Ray.

One night, a week or two later, Ray awakened me, talking loudly, almost yelling in his sleep. He was in such distress, I woke him up. He told me that he dreamed we were in France long ago and that there was fighting and disorder all about. He said that we had been in the bedroom, then described the large, dark, four-poster bed with heavy curtains around it. He said we had been very happy there, but clearly in his dream he had not been tuned in to my resentment and hurt feelings. Then he described my long golden gown and said that we were getting ready to retire for the night when he heard loud banging on the downstairs door. There was much chaos, fighting, looting, and burning going on in the city. It was a very dangerous time and he was afraid of burglars. He heard the banging on the doors, so he went downstairs and took his long sword with him.

He remembered that he had on a loose white shirt, black pants and boots, his hair was longer, and he had a beard. When he got downstairs, a group of thieves was trying to break in, and he was fending them off with his sword. I had awakened him during the battle. I listened to his dream in amazement, then reached over into my nightstand drawer, took the written page with my dream on it, and showed it to him. He was amazed at what I had written. We agreed that this couldn't be a coincidence.

It probably shouldn't have surprised me, because I've had a number of conscious recalls and dreams from what I felt were former lives. Ray's dream confirmed mine and I was delighted. However, Ray was puzzled. He couldn't explain it. All he could say to me was, "Well, maybe there's something to it after all." I realized then that we were still working on communication in this lifetime. We could never get on the same wavelength when it came to heart-to-heart intimacy, and at that time I just didn't know what to do about it. I was tired of trying to explain what I needed from him.

When we arrived for our conference with the oncologist, we learned that Ray had had a good night and had slept well. The girls and I gathered to wait in the hospital solarium, and Dr. Thomas appeared on time. He was a large man who moved with an uncanny birdlike agility and swiftness. In one darting sweep, his light brown eyes took us all in. He seated himself at a round table, adjusted his glasses on his hawk-like nose, and motioned us to join him. He had Ray's chart in front of him and proceeded to review it, explaining the surgery and Ray's condition from a medical point of view. Cindy rapidly fired questions at him, but he could not answer them as quickly as she asked them. He pulled back from the table as though under attack and good-naturedly held up his hands in mock defense. Then he leaned forward, taking the questions one at a time. There were four of us, so we had verbally overwhelmed him.

"This type of cancer is extremely aggressive, not common, and unpredictable," he said. He gave us the name of the cancer, and I thought it must have contained every letter of the alphabet: "Peritoneal carcinomatosis, secondary to metastatic mucinous adenocarcinoma." He reviewed the drug therapy program he had worked up, stating that it was imperative that Ray get started on chemotherapy immediately.

He continued, "Everyone reacts differently both emotionally and physically to the drug therapy. Some of the hardest-working, positive patients don't make it, while the most miserable, contrary people with negative attitudes are successful. I don't know why."

He told us that the chemo treatment had a 20-40 percent recovery record with minimal side effects. It was hoped that this would shrink the tumors and dry up the fluid that they excrete. "There is always hope," he said. "Never, never give up hope." He was positive and allowed us a brief smile. The treatment would be administered twice a month—three times the first month.

We stared at him silently for a few minutes while we tried to assimilate all this information. I knew there would be many more questions later, but right then we couldn't process any more information. Our minds were on overload.

I asked him about visualization therapy to help Ray heal himself and shrink the cancerous tumors. In this type of therapy, the patient visualizes his white cells destroying the cancer cells.

"Yes," he said. "I know about this. Of course, I have no objection to using this along with drug therapy." I would ask Ray first if he wanted to try it, then speak with Annmarie and John, who used visualization in their work.

Dr. Thomas hadn't realized then how much his own positive attitude had helped us. Or perhaps he did. He said he wanted to check the pathological report and confirm what the surgeon had eyeballed during surgery. He also wanted to talk with Ray, "alone."

We all stayed in the solarium, wandering about aimlessly, picking up magazines that we really didn't see and staring out the windows at the movement of traffic crawling along the highway below. Betsy was standing halfway out the door and was the first to see Dr. Thomas exit Ray's room. She rushed down the corridor to her dad and had a minute with him before we collected ourselves and joined her.

She told me later that he had tears in his eyes and was quite shaken when she entered his room. He had asked her, "Does Mom know?" She had told him yes, and a minute later we all walked in. It only took him that minute to compose himself somewhat for us, but from that moment on his pale drawn face would be indelibly stamped on my memory. Perhaps that was one of the hardest and most painful moments of all for me. I would have given anything to have spared him that span of minutes. I felt such pain in my heart that it actually seemed physical. It was a moment of complete helplessness for all of us, and I felt captured by the silent spreading invader. The feeling was overwhelming and complete, triggering thoughts of my horrendous dream of the gigantic snake which had seized Ray. In my dream of last August, the snake turned into an octopus. The memory was vivid, but I still wasn't sure what it meant.

I felt him withdrawing from us as we hugged and kissed him, then stood silently waiting for him to speak. The silence continued, and I just couldn't stand it. "What did the doctor tell you?" I asked. His inner dam broke, the words pouring forth, and he told us, almost verbatim, the complete conversation he had had with the doctor. Ray told me Dr. Thomas had been very truthful. "I asked him if I was going to die," he said soberly, adding, "and I asked him when."

I felt as if I couldn't breathe. If it were I, would I be this courageous and come right to the point? I didn't know. Then Ray continued, "He said he couldn't predict the future. He had no answers. I asked him if I had a chance, and he told me there is always a chance." Then with confidence, Ray said, "I told him I wanted to go ahead with the chemo."

I knew immediately that Dr. Thomas had conveyed the single most important factor to Ray—that of hope. Hope had been presented positively and clearly. I saw the determined set of Ray's mouth, the slight, but positive rise of his shoulders against the pillows, and the resolved expression on his face. I looked closely at him and knew he had grabbed onto something. But how long he would be able to hold on to this new hope was another question. I didn't want to think about it.

Exhaustion soon overcame him, and he wanted to sleep. I could feel his weariness; we had talked enough. Emotions hung raw, clinging to the very air and seeming to fill up the space in the room. They vibrated around us and transformed themselves into waves of feeling. I knew that he wanted to be alone, that it was time for us to leave. Lou and Annmarie were coming tomorrow to pray with us, and I reminded Ray of that as I hugged him good-night.

I mentioned that Dr. Thomas had no objection to visualization therapy and asked him how he felt about it. He was agreeable to trying visualization, but told me he would be more comfortable starting a program after he got home. I was pleased and surprised that he had agreed so easily and wondered how it would work out. I considered visualization therapy a metaphysical process, and I had never before asked Ray to join in any kind of experience like that. I wondered how he had so easily changed his status from observer to participant.

In the light of Ray's horrible diagnosis, I clung to my inner truths for sustenance. My inner spiritual foundation remained firm and constant, but a great chasm began to form between my emotional humanness and my inner spirit. I felt that the only way to bridge this gap was to surrender and trust in God, but I wondered, in the months ahead, if I would be able to do that without reservation.

On the morning of the third day after surgery, I arrived early at the hospital and learned that Ray had had a good night—at least physically. But he was emotionally depressed that morning, and I didn't know what to do to help him. The thought of how I would react to all this flew across my mind again, and I couldn't stand it. Then, without words, Ray conveyed to me that he needed his own space and wanted to be alone. I desperately wanted to help him, but I couldn't. I knew I had to step back and give him the room he needed. I loved him so dearly that my heart was hurting, but I was not able to take this terrible trial away from him.

My tears started again, but I didn't want to break down. I wanted to try to move on into the line of battle, out of the valley of shadows where I felt so helpless. I never thought there was anything wrong with crying. Weeping is an emotional release and cleansing, but I knew I couldn't just sit and cry all the time. It was upsetting to Ray; he didn't need that. I felt so frustrated that I could do little more than go downstairs and have a cup of tea.

I had made arrangements with Annmarie and her friend Lou to meet me at the hospital later that morning to help me pray for Ray. Lou worked in the field of education and had been ordained as a minister through the Movement of Spiritual Inner Awareness (M.S.I.A.), based in Los Angeles. His philosophy of life seemed to align closely in many ways with mine, so it was comforting to have him there.

He led us in forming a prayer circle around Ray's bed in what turned out to be a beautiful, energy-filled visualization experience. As we stood together, Lou called forth the Holy Spirit. He asked that the light of the Holy Spirit surround and protect us, and also that Ray would receive the light for his highest good—emotionally, physically, and spiritually. Lou then guided us not to expect any particular results, but to let the Holy Spirit do God's will. He asked us to help by mentally visualizing the light Ray was receiving. He led us as we pictured huge pillars of white light, building them tall and strong in the four corners of the room. Then we called for spiritual strength and positive energy from God to fill Ray, and we prayed for His help. Lou asked Ray to look up to the light and let it in—he told him that that's all he had to do.

Then Lou joined us in silent meditation for awhile, and we all sensed the radiant energy fill up the room. After Lou finished, Ray told him that he felt peaceful and rested, and thanked Lou for coming. As for me, I was grateful to have such close supportive friends.

Later in the day, Ray became terribly despondent again. He was disinterested in conversation, detached, and lost in his own thoughts. I tried to break through but after an attempt at trivial talk, I gave up. There was nothing I could do. I only hoped that my presence was helping somehow. I realized that he was grappling with an enormous emotional trauma, and that his normal reaction would be depression. I was also aware that at times he really didn't want us around. I wasn't hurt by this because I knew the situation was overwhelming him. I wasn't sure how the girls felt, but none of us were able to stay away for any long stretches of time. We raced back and forth between home and hospital and just couldn't bear to leave him.

Gloom hung in the air that evening—thick, dark, and oppressive—and I wished I could sweep it clean with a brush of bright, etheric light. Finally, we decided it was time to leave. To make matters worse, the girls and I were getting touchy among ourselves. Afterward we had a long talk, though nothing we said made anything better. It was just too awful; Ray was too young to leave us. That thought was constantly on our minds.

On the fourth day after surgery, Ray was better in some ways physically, but he was not ready to eat anything. He told me not to come until 2:30 in the afternoon. When I arrived, my spirits were lifted when I saw that he had shaved and changed into fresh pajamas. Shortly after I got there, his younger brother Johnny arrived with Grandma Eva. He had driven down from upstate New York and stopped on his way to pick her up. John was so crushed when he saw Ray that he had to stand in the hall to compose himself. His tears flowed freely, and he couldn't speak.

Johnny had always shown emotion more openly than Ray, and he was overcome. The brothers were so different; they didn't even resemble each other physically. While Ray was tall and dark, with fair skin and hazel eyes, Johnny was short and baby-faced. Ray was like his mother, carefully guarded and frequently censoring his conversation with others. He had never been intimately spontaneous and hid his emotions. His dry wit and outward sociability led others to believe they knew him well, but most never really got past the exterior level. His engineering background only grounded him in logic and further amplified this analytical inward demeanor.

I had been married to him for thirty-three years, but I still had not broken completely into his inner recesses. Over the years I had tried continually and had definitely gained a lot of ground. But Ray guarded his inner psyche carefully; I felt that I would never fully know his heart. That thought had always made me sad. I fervently wished that at some place in our togetherness he would find a way to open himself completely to me. But after thirty-three years, I had just about come to accept the reality, though I knew I would still keep trying.

John was very much like their father, high strung and emotional. Ray's father, John, Sr., was raised under the influence of his parents, first-generation Italian immigrants. The grandfather had learned English shortly after he arrived in the United States, but the grandmother, after living here fifty years, still spoke only Italian. The grandfather was the patriarch; domineering, self-centered, and macho. This was passed onto Ray's father, where it took root. His father had been an alcoholic, as was his father before him, and was abusive to the family. He really led his own life, living with the family but apart. Ray learned early to suppress any conversation that would cause the slightest offense to his father. This conditioned self-censorship, I felt, had contributed to Ray's inability to communicate spontaneously throughout his life.

Ray worked from sixth grade on, delivering telegrams for Western Union on his bicycle. It allowed him to pursue flying lessons while he was in high school and to receive his private pilot's license. Being a Sagittarian, he always had the wanderlust; at fourteen he traveled the New York subway system extensively by himself. His mother's father had been a train engineer on the Erie-Lackawanna Railroad, and Ray became an expert on that system, too. His early love of trains continued his entire life.

Because of his difficult home life, Ray joined the air force when he was seventeen after graduating from high school. We met in 1952 through a mutual acquaintance when he was home on leave. I had started college in the Midwest with the dream of becoming a journalist, but found I was really not prepared in many ways—among them, I lacked self-discipline. I dropped out in 1952 to try to discover where I was going in life. The attraction we felt for each other was strong and immediate. He had such an air of freedom about him, and I gravitated powerfully toward his philosophy that nothing in life was impossible to achieve. Ray had a magnetic charisma about him and put forth a strong masculine presence. People reacted to his air of confidence, but most of the time he was unaware of the effect he had on them. I was amazed at his naivete. When I kidded him about this quality, he would say, "You're crazy," and become embarrassed.

I was raised in a strict Catholic home ruled by an overly domineering religious father. I knew my father loved me as well as my brother and sister, but he was so shackled by his beliefs that they ruled supreme. His single rebellious act in life had been to marry my long-suffering mother who was a Presbyterian. I admired her for never relinquishing her own religion for him. My mother's beliefs softened my strict Catholic upbringing, a fact I only realized later in life.

When I told my parents that I wanted to marry Ray, my father forbade me, saying I was only nineteen and too young. There was to be no discussion about it, so Ray and I eloped in April of 1953 and were married by a justice of the peace. Ray was legally under age and had to have a note from his mother, which would be a running joke our entire married life. I left my father's house in disgrace and settled in Great Falls, Montana, where Ray had been assigned his remaining two years in the air force. My father refused to speak to us or have any contact with us until we were married by a priest six months later at the base chapel in Montana.

We visited home that Christmas of 1953. Two weeks later, after we had returned to Montana, my father suffered a severe coronary and died two days later. I have always thanked God that we were given the opportunity to make our peace with him.

My father's funeral was on a cold, bleak, snowy day in January. The huge church was filled to capacity. That entire year had been traumatic for me; I was close to hysteria, so Ray took me outside the church. I asked for a sign that I had been truly forgiven by my father and that he was at peace. While we stood in the vestibule and waited, the pall bearers brought the coffin back out and set the casket down near me for a moment to open the church doors. As I silently spoke to my father, a radiant beam of sunshine broke through the overcast gray sky, piercing the round church window above the casket. The light struck the metal cross on the coffin, illuminating the entire casket with such a brilliant light that I brought my hand up to protect my eyes. I looked up at the window, and the overcast gray sky was evident again. Relief and thankfulness washed over me that my father was at peace.

After Ray's discharge from the air force, we left for Indiana, where Ray attended four years of college and where Cindy was born in 1956. It was a hard four years; Cindy was an infant, and Ray was working two part-time jobs. I still see him persistently bending over his books, dead tired and calling to me to put the coffee on. In 1958 Ray received his degree in electronics engineering. We went back home then to Rockland County, New York. In 1960 and 1961, respectively, Betsy and Holly were born in Nyack.

From 1964 on, Ray was working in the space program, and we moved frequently—living in Alabama, Chicago, Florida, and finally back to the East to give the kids some stability, settling permanently in Pennsylvania in 1972. I loved living in different areas of the country, and it allowed us to really appreciate the life styles of other sections of the United States. We lived in Florida for seven years, where our youngest daughter Gina was born and when the space program was in full bloom.

Cindy remembers standing in the school yard with her classmates, watching the huge rockets being launched. Ray was acquainted with a few of the astronauts at that time. They would occasionally call him and ask if he would like to fly "down range" with them in their huge jets. He couldn't get out the door fast enough. He loved being "on the edge" in everything he did. Ray had qualified for the air force cadet program during his first year in the service when he was single, but had given it up when we married. I often wondered whether he had regretted missing his chance to fly the big jets, even though he denied it. More than once he said to me, "If I could have one wish, I'd be in the astronaut program."

Ray's own flying had been frequent, in small planes, and he had even received his instructor's license. His love of flying continued throughout his life. It was the freedom of soaring above the earth that he loved so much, the feeling of being free of physical confinement. I looked at Ray that day and thought how after all these years together, I still found him to be such a private person, who never actually put his own philosophy of life into words.

Several days later, Ray reached a turning point and continued to improve. I was amazed that his body could sustain such a traumatic invasion and then rally so rapidly. His spirits were climbing, they carried us along, and I found that I could still smile.

Chapter Three

TAKING FLIGHT

(January 20-21)

At the hospital Social Services program, we were asked if we needed any information or guidance. We felt we could use all the help that was available, so that afternoon we sat down with a counselor. However, after receiving her onslaught of negative remarks and advice, we thanked her and left.

Amazingly, as we moved into the front line of battle with Ray's cancer, we found that to many counselors maintaining hope is synonymous with denying reality. Many of those with whom we spoke took the immediate approach that we were denying the unavoidability of Ray's death, which put us in the difficult position of feeling hopeless. It was clear to all of us that more counselors need to weigh everything they hear and listen to families more carefully.

In life and death situations, theory is dry and offensive, and textbook advice often unacceptable. We found, surprisingly, that the medical staff had a more positive attitude than the counselors. We had to move ahead for Ray's sake and didn't want to feel that we had to constantly defend our feelings of hope.

I now felt strongly that, in this situation, hope and faith were synonymous. While studying Edgar Cayce's readings, I remembered learning that faith is an attribute of the soul. Faith may be denied or renounced until it ceases to exist within the consciousness, or it can be exercised until it can move mountains. But I learned that day that faith has different meanings to different people.

Cayce sometimes said in his readings to be careful what you ask for—you might get it! Yet, I came to believe that faith means the ability to put an event or situation into the hands of God. I accepted that the soul is the best judge of its own journey. I believed without the slightest doubt that Ray's soul possessed the wisdom of God, but I didn't have the vision at that time to see how his journey might have led to this sickness. I finally acknowledged how angry and frustrated I was, but I also admitted that there was nothing I could do about it. I knew I had to listen to what God was telling me inside and also to have faith that He was with Ray, that the outcome would be the most beneficial to his soul—whatever it was to be. The most monumental task for me would be to accept God's solution.

I resolved that this was where my faith had to start. I decided to give everything over to God, but I also asked His help to do so. Strange as it seemed, however, as soon as I started to surrender, even a little bit, it helped me to know that someone else was in charge. It wasn't easy, and it didn't happen in a flash because there was a wide gap between where my emotional self wanted to take me and what I was trying to accomplish in spirit. Gradually, as my surrendering continued a little at a time, the Holy Spirit began to send answers along the way: conscious encounters with God's universe and His compassionate heart.

Ray would be coming home soon, and we wanted to get a visualization program worked out. Cindy picked up a marvelous book that Annmarie and John used in their programs. After I read it, I was impressed with the results that the author had achieved. *Getting Well Again,* by Carl Simonton (Bantam

Books, 1978), is a wonderful book, which I would recommend to anyone interested in visualization therapy. I brought it to the hospital, and Ray read it, too. He was excited with what the book had to say, and I was relieved. It gave us all a good overall explanation of how visualization therapy works. I believed very strongly in the power of visualization, and still do today.

The goal of such therapy for cancer patients is to find some meaningful way to visualize the cancer cells being destroyed. The therapy must be programmed for each patient individually because the operative symbols will be different for different people. An important benefit of visualization is that it allows cancer patients to actively participate in their own healing. It's a way in which they can begin to fight their illness on a mental level. This was very important to Ray. He felt he had lost all control over what was happening to his body.

Cayce himself was a strong believer in the powers of visualization. In reading 3577-1 he said, "Then, spiritualize and visualize purposes, in the manner in which the entity desires things to be done, and you'll have them done!" Only time would tell what visualization could achieve for Ray.

Annmarie and her husband John offered to work up a specific program for Ray to use when he got home. On his behalf, Annmarie spoke to another doctor who worked extensively in this field. She also spoke to Ray's surgeon, asking him for specific details of what he had seen during surgery so she could incorporate it into the visualization. Sadly, she hadn't realized the extent of the cancer invasion, so when he told her, she was very upset. She had great faith, though, and didn't doubt the occurrence of miracles. She wanted to get one started immediately, and I was totally uplifted by her optimism.

Ray was extremely positive about the upcoming chemotherapy. His belief system strongly incorporated advanced medical technology. He explained to me that the chemo drug uses "a search and destroy" method—something to which an air force man could relate. Dr. Thomas told him that the results had been good with other cancer patients and that he had a good chance. I prayed that his belief system would be strong enough to carry him through and that the chemotherapy drug would achieve results.

It was around that time that Annmarie offered to channel information for us from a spirit entity named "Josef." In 1986, there were many varied opinions about channeling, and I still didn't know what I believed. It seemed reasonable to me that channeled information came from the channeler's higher self or spiritual consciousness—that deep inner core still connected to our essence that dwelled with God or our kingdom within.

Edgar Cayce, who gave readings while "asleep," had his own thoughts about where the information came from. In the book, *Edgar Cayce on ESP* (Warner Books, 1969), author Doris Agee relates Cayce's description of the levels of the unconscious mind. He talked about the collective unconscious, in which the individual unconscious has its origin. This collective, or universal, unconscious he described as a vast "river" of thought flowing through eternity, fed by the collective mental activity of humankind since its beginning.

According to Cayce, this collective unconscious is accessible to all who develop their own psychic faculties to such a degree as to be able to draw from, as well as feed into, this river of thought. In the light of Ray's illness, I wanted to use every resource available to him. Annmarie had been channeling for a number of years, and my daughters and I had received numerous readings from her. When Annmarie went into trance, she took on the demeanor of an older gentleman; very firm, kindly, and with a dry sense of humor. The information was always helpful, positive, and spiritual with a high degree of accuracy. I remembered Ray sitting in the den, listening intently to prior readings. Now he was anxious to hear what information Josef could offer him. A short time later we listened to the tape. Josef had said the following during the reading:

Well, he is doing just fine. That is the important thing to remember here. He is just fine. What happens to a physical body is of no importance to the spirit, and it is important to realize that. It is also important to realize that where there is breath, there is hope and that anything on the planet can be lifted to the light with sufficient faith and a good attitude.

Now this is a time for Raymond [Josef always called him that] to search within himself to find the God within; not to pray to some god in the sky, but to look within—to know that who he is is eternal. That something such as cancer is a very insignificant little bug and can be squashed or can be used for his benefit and his growth. And this is a time for tremendous growth for him; tremendous growth. He can use it to become one with God again.

He got caught up a little bit too much in the physical dense world, and this is the way his soul has decided to pull himself out. Now as far as life expectancy, that is up to him. He'll make the choice as he goes along—not a conscious choice; he'll make it in the dream state with his higher self, and he will make that decision depending on what is the highest good for everyone concerned.

Where is the most growth? Is it in fighting this disease? Is it in overcoming it or succumbing to it? Will Jan [my nickname] become independent, regardless of which way it goes, and will the children search for faith instead of looking to medical science to save what is in God's hands to begin with?

Josef went on to say that, on a physical level, Ray should exercise when able. He also advised that homeopathic remedies be taken in conjunction with traditional medicine to boost his immune system and lessen the negative side effects of the drugs. There should be no intake of meat, only white fish but no shellfish. Many grains should be taken, such as millet and oat bran, oat bran being good for the blood. He was to eat lots of fiber and four vegetables per day, two taken raw and two partially cooked. He suggested papaya, and that it could be taken dried. He was to eliminate sugar and caffeine, but have some honey. His vitamin supplements should consist of minerals, especially manganese and selenium, a high content of Vitamin A, and some form of beta carotene and E in high dosages with an added supplement of lethicin and kelp.

Josef continued, pressing on into the sensitive area of Ray's spiritual life:

> Emotionally, he ought to be down on his hands and knees praying for guidance. By getting on your knees, you are placing emphasis on understanding. And he should not ask for life because that is always given, but for acceptance and guidance and strength. As to his family, they would do well to appreciate what they have in a father, in a husband, and it is a time not for grief but for appreciation. And that is all I have to say for the moment.

He said he would give more information in about two weeks. Ray found it most interesting that Josef had suggested that his soul really hadn't made a choice yet. He looked at me closely. "Well, at least he didn't say I was going to die."

Ray felt that the philosophical content of Josef's message rang true, and I agreed. However, I was concerned about the menu suggested because Ray had always been a picky eater. He was stubborn and unreasonable about his choices of food.

He wanted to think about the reading more. He did say he was going to try the foods suggested as soon as he was home.

The days began to blend together. At times it seemed I had lived a lifetime in a little more than two weeks, and I kept looking back to only a month before when everything was fine. A feeling of unreality was constantly with me, and I functioned in a dreamlike state. I seemed to be always waiting to wake up. Our lives were now focused on hospital visits, medical terminology, and Ray's progress. It preoccupied us day and night, invaded our dreams, turned everything into tunnel vision, with the tunnel always being the path to the hospital.

The sixth night after surgery I was in bed trying to fall asleep. Quietly and unobtrusively around midnight, an uncanny feeling of peace flowed into my room. I felt bathed in white, yellow, and pink lights. For the first time in a very long while, tension slipped out of my body, and order and harmony quietly replaced anxiety. Although I wondered what was happening, I welcomed it with an open heart. As the calmness spread throughout my body, an image of Ray was imprinted in my mind, which I could not understand. I thought I must ask him in the morning if anything unusual was happening to him around this time of night. I was later rewarded with a sound night's sleep.

Ray called early the next morning, and I asked him immediately if he had had any dreams last night, and he laughed.

"Did I dream?" he whispered into the phone. "I'm not sure, but you won't believe what happened to me last night."

He wouldn't part with any more information until I saw him, so he asked me to hurry over. He sounded very excited. I couldn't imagine what had happened. Wondering what it was all about, I quickly dressed and drove to the hospital.

He was sitting up in bed when I walked into the room, and immediately, without even a greeting, he again said to me, "You're not going to believe me when I tell you this."

I assured him that absolutely nothing was beyond my belief at that point. Then he began to tell me about a strange experience he'd had the night before. He was on the verge of falling asleep when he experienced the sensation of his bed suddenly shaking violently. It then started moving toward the door and out into the hall. He saw himself in the bed, yet he was above the bed watching it all. He was very frightened, so he sat up quickly, an action which stopped the movement of the bed.

He thought to himself, beds just don't move by themselves! He settled down, not understanding what was happening because *he was awake*. It happened again, but this time he found himself in the bed going down the hall, watching himself. For a second time he pulled himself back to full alertness, but was becoming curious as to what would happen if he would just let it continue. Three times he settled himself; each time the bed started to shake. But now, he said, his curiosity had triumphed. He decided to go with it.

Out the door, into the hall he moved, riding in the bed, hearing the wheels clickety-clacking as the bed traveled swiftly over the white square tiles in the hall; glaring overhead lights whizzing by. He saw all this as though he were out of his body and found it most interesting. The pace was fast, and within seconds the bed had wheeled him into another room.

"I saw bright light coming in through the windows," he said, "and the whole room was lit up like daytime from the light. The nurse was there who came to see me this afternoon. She's the one who will be doing the chemo. Doctor Thomas was there, too. It seemed I was in some kind of a therapy room, and there were bottles hanging here and there on stands and different medical equipment all around. Then the doctor turned to me and said, 'Let's hit a home run!' "

With a jolt, Ray found himself back in his room, unable to understand what had happened. "It wasn't a dream," he emphasized repeatedly. As soon as he finished, I knew that he had had an "out-of-body" experience, which can happen in times of great physical or emotional stress, and he'd certainly had his share of both. It was a startling, emotionally moving event for him that didn't happen to everyone. When it does occur, many aren't fortunate enough to remember it that clearly.

Ray declared adamantly that he had not been asleep; he had taken no drugs and he was in a very comfortable relaxed state. Perhaps this was the assurance he needed during this trauma that there *is* something else besides the physical body. I remembered that Lou had said to him during our prayer communion, "Just let the light in," and he did. He told me he found the trip extremely exciting. Once he had decided to go with it, he lost his fear of it. Annmarie said later it was incredible that he had recalled the trip so vividly. Ray's conscious encounters with spirit had begun, and this was to be the first of many.

The doctors decided to proceed with the chemotherapy, and the first session was completed right away in his room. We were elated that everything went well and that he experienced only minor side effects. We didn't give his strange experience another thought during the next several days.

A week later, Ray learned that he would be taken to another room for his second treatment. To his amazement, he found himself in the same room he had visited the night of his out-of-body experience. He said that, when they wheeled him into the room, he thought seriously about telling them that he'd been there before. He felt quite comfortable and was dumbfounded to see that the room was exactly as he had seen it that night. The windows were where he had seen them, as were the beds and chairs. One chair was missing, and he asked the nurse where the chair was that had been there. She told him they had moved it that morning. His oncologist was present as well as the same nurse—all exactly as he had seen them.

Ray went into that chemotherapy treatment unafraid and positive. The nurse remarked to him that she wished they could "bottle his attitude." He felt sad that he couldn't share the event with both of them, but he feared ridicule or an accusation of hallucinating. His higher self had made use of his astral body to help him allay the fear and apprehension of the chemotherapy by showing him beforehand what would happen. It lifted his spirits and proved again, strongly, that there was much more to life than what he could physically see and feel.

Twelve days after surgery, we were finally going to bring Ray home. Those past days had seemed endless; time seemed to be always playing tricks with my mind. For me, the relentless feeling of unreality continued, and my dream-like state persevered. I could not deny the present by allowing myself to project into a created future, nor by detaching myself into a dream world. How could I live in the present when part of my mind did not want to accept what was happening? Where was I in my own life?

A foggy opaque mist had descended, and I was treading in its swirling grayness. I was sick and tired of people telling me "one day at a time." I didn't want each day. I was groping around in that swirling grayness, feeling trapped and guilty about feeling trapped. After all, I was the one with the spiritual awareness. Despite what I "knew" deep down inside, it didn't help my emotional self. I felt I really had no choices; that's a terrible realization. "You can give it back to God and ask spirit for help," an inner voice kept insisting. I asked how I could do this completely and reminded my inner voice to remember that I was only human. But there was no answer.

When I arrived at the hospital the next morning, Dr. Thomas was in Ray's room finishing his examination. I helped Ray to get dressed; he was so anxious to leave. Evidently Ray had caught a cold or virus, which had just started to surface that day. The doctor was concerned and wanted to keep him in the hospital another day, but Ray was so insistent on leaving that he released him. After I took care of the check-out bureaucracy, we pushed through the lobby doors and out into another overcast gray day. As we felt the slight warmth of a faded January sun, a quick fantasy skipped across my mind: we had left all the horror behind us in that huge caretaker of a building. But I knew it was only that physical separation from the hospital that prompted the thought.

Ray brought medicine home with him—more antibiotics. The coughing started again, making him uncomfortable, weak, and miserable. His body and emotions had been completely invaded. I had no idea how he would deal with such trauma, much less put it into any kind of perspective. His first night home was a restless one for him and a scary one for me. I was frightened to be alone with him, concerned that something might happen and I wouldn't know what to do. His surgery wound had not yet healed, and there was a drain protruding from his abdomen.

When morning came, I welcomed the sunlight creeping in through the blinds, ending a long, worry-filled night. When we awoke, I discovered that a new and growing depression had surfaced in Ray. Erratic mood swings would become a pattern throughout the weeks to come. I sensed he was overwhelmed and needed time to sort it all out. I didn't know how he was going to come to terms with it all, when I couldn't even grasp the reality of it myself or imagine what thoughts were running through his head. I had no idea how I could help him. My love for him could only present itself as support; I was devastated because I hadn't the ability to help him relieve the mental anguish or the physical discomfort. He was totally into himself, even turning his face away from me. This time I had no verbal probes or feelers to use to break through. What could I say to him? So, I left him alone to give him some time.

In the afternoon a few days later, I was sitting on the bed

near him, when spontaneous weeping overcame me. Ray put his arms around me and tried to assure me that he would get well, but somehow my sobs triggered a reaction in him that caused his words to suddenly spill out to me like a tap turned on full. He told me he had been depressed for a very long time—even before his illness. I had been aware of that, but not to the extent he was confessing now. I remembered the last year and a half and how difficult it had been for him when he was laid off without warning by a large impersonal company.

Ray had been an electronics engineer involved in the design and marketing of sophisticated telephone systems to large corporations. Although he was a maverick and marched to his own drummer, his brilliant inventiveness and charisma in business made him a valuable asset. He had proven his abilities, although sometimes unconventionally, so he was usually given the "impossible" assignments. He enjoyed his job tremendously and was always an enthusiastic worker. He hadn't been singled out; his whole group and thousands of others had fallen prey to the layoff. But this wasn't much comfort to him.

He had done private consulting after the layoff and had just recently been hired by a small, newly formed company when he got sick. He had seemed so happy and had tried to be enthused about the new job. He kept telling me he would be able to "do his own thing" in this small corporation. But it was a big cut in salary and the benefits were nowhere near what we had had before. The loss of his former job was a terrible blow to him. I was sure it was much more of a loss than he had allowed himself to express.

We had both assumed that his former job would take him through to retirement. We kept telling ourselves that any problems concerning finances, moving, and his new job would eventually be resolved. However, I had felt that his reserve of optimism was overtaxed, that it might take him a long time to recover. Ray had great reserves of energy and his flexibility was extraordinary, but I wondered what he did with all that unexpressed anger.

"What are you doing with your anger?" I would ask him time and time again. I tried to get him to express his rage, because I felt that emotions created by an event should be expressed or they would stay with you; but he would not. Looking back, I sensed that he had never fully recovered from the depression he felt over the layoff, no matter what he had said. The past few years had also brought many changes in the family: marriages and divorces, new grandchildren, and we had both reached our midlife of fifty years old, yet we had all managed to come out the other side in one piece.

It took hard work, support, consideration, tenacity, and unconditional love for each of us to weather these storms together. It also took a bit of trusting ourselves. The love, closeness, and being there for each other had been the foundation for each of us to grow and follow our own path in life.

There had been a few rules that I followed in rearing my daughters. Unconditional love had always been first. To love someone on your terms was not my definition of love. That's how I had been raised. It's easy to love kids who aren't boat-rockers, but ours were real shakers, and shakers test you daily. Children are never stamped out by cookie cutters, neither are they extensions of their parents. Children are entities unto themselves, with their own souls, who eventually would be responsible for themselves. As Edgar Cayce said in reading 811-2: " . . . each soul must find its *own* impulse, its *own* ideal." Ray also had this belief, without putting it into so many words, and we were proud of our daughters and loved them very much. Still, it was easier for us to maintain unconditional love for our children than it was for ourselves.

Given the stresses of the past few years and then the loss of Ray's job, perhaps the shock had been considerably more than he had been able to handle. As I recalled these impressions, I realized that his depression had started soon after that, but because of his frequent withdrawals into himself, it made it difficult for me to grasp the depth of his depression. As I remembered, his mood was up and down for a few months after the layoff, then he seemed to level off. Perhaps he felt defeated and his longtime reservoir of energy and enthusiasm had been short-circuited. Perhaps his reserves had been used up on other trials in life that he had faced squarely—about which I knew little or nothing.

Now I was finally hearing him express the deepest parts of himself, and my heart just wept. His quiet strength had always kept him a private person, even to me, but now I was learning how very depressed he'd been—how he'd kept the truth to himself, thinking there was no real answer. It seemed that the depression had magnified all his insecurities and that the loss of his "secure" job had trapped him in a professional and personal void. In this depression, he had bombarded himself with negative thoughts of being unloved and uncared for by the family, although he then told me he knew deep down that these thoughts weren't true. I wondered how much of these feelings came from his being an observer so much of the time instead of a participant, never allowing himself to become fully integrated into the family group.

The extent of his emotional downfall had been huge and overwhelming, but he said he thought he could handle it. Instead of reaching out to me, he retreated more deeply inside.

Now he told me, "I just have to change my way of thinking. It's very important. What I've been feeling isn't true." He confessed that he felt badly then about doubting our love and caring, but I told him it was all right and that maybe something inside him *needed* to feel that way. He wondered why he needed proof of our love, why he didn't just know that we loved him. He now realized our deep concern for him and that we were there for him. He told me he knew he must rid himself of all these doubts, but he needed our help. "I can't change overnight," he sighed.

I couldn't stop sobbing; we only wanted to hold and comfort each other, which we did. I beat myself up for a long time after that, angry that I had not been fully aware of the depth of his depression the previous year.

"Just let the light in," I whispered, and he nodded.

Many personal feelings were discussed that day and brought out into the open. It was like a cleansing and purging for him. Although I didn't understand the whys of it all, at least it was finally being expressed and I had been able to dispel some of his fears. Evidently it had relieved him a great deal, so this new opening began to bring about a rapid, dramatic change in him.

Miraculously, his appetite increased. He started getting up, dressing, and coming downstairs. He resumed his traditional morning trips to the 7-11 store for that first cup of coffee. Images came to my mind of the kids when they were little, running out the door in their pajamas to accompany Daddy on his early morning run to the 7-11. Later, he wanted to start doing some work at home as his physical ability permitted.

But soon the anxiety of fulfilling new job demands began to bother him. I wished badly that money wasn't such an issue for us so he wouldn't have to worry about his job. As his cold cleared up with the help of the antibiotics, he felt better and started to become much more positive about his healing. We planned to start the visualization program as soon as he was ready. I had not pushed him on this.

The next doctor's appointment was uplifting. His progress had been good, and Dr. Thomas remarked that a tragic situation was turning out well. The grin on Ray's face confirmed his own attitude. Later, at the surgeon's office, it was the same story. Very much a realist, the surgeon was extremely pleased with Ray's progress. He smiled and said, "So you decided to beat it, huh?"

It seemed to be an important turning point.

A few days later, Gina was picking Ray up after his chemotherapy treatment. He had finished early and was waiting for her in the solarium. Gina walked past the door and didn't realize it was her father silently sitting there, staring out the large window. He told her he had been deep in thought, visualizing his stomach and what was going on inside. This introspection surprised me because we had not started a visualization program yet. He had been reading some of my books over the past several weeks, but I didn't know if that was making any impact. Ray's new attitude included not only becoming more verbal but also somewhat demanding. His good progress continued, and the doctors were pleased. I was ecstatic!

One night shortly afterward, I came into the bedroom at midnight to give him his pills. I found him awake, waiting to talk. Being much more outspoken was one of his new goals, he informed me, and I was to prepare myself for it. His curiosity had been peaked by his astral experience in the hospital bed and made him hungry for more knowledge about it. He finally began to express his deeper thoughts and questions about psychic ability, telling me for the first time in our thirty-three years of marriage that he had always had this tool, though he said that he felt he had never used it correctly. I was more surprised by the fact that he was expressing this, than by the fact that he had this ability.

I had known for years that it was routine for him to dream a solution to a business predicament or even the answer to a complicated technical problem. He'd receive the answer while he was sleeping, get up in the middle of the night, and write down the solution. His uncanny sense of direction was phenomenal; I felt it was more than instinct. He always knew who was on the phone or where someone had left something. He never lost a thing of his own. He was an excellent sender in our family telepathic connection. Combined with these inner assets, he had a photographic memory and an extremely high I.Q.

After much reflection, he realized what an asset psychic ability could be and what tremendous help it could offer in choosing the right direction in life. He felt he had made many decisions that he knew inherently were incorrect, based on emotion. He didn't know why he had rejected the inside wisdom and information and thought perhaps it was because it had no basis in fact—that it wasn't tangible. He told me he had not been ready to depend upon the information coming from his inner self. Now he wanted to experience it fully and was not afraid to try to listen to his inner self. "I want to go to church this Sunday," he said, "and get down on my knees and pray."

I was suddenly filled with joy, thinking perhaps that this was the right time for me to begin living in the present.

Ray had mentioned to me that he had regretted not having more routine medical checkups. His yearly pilot's physical was not complete enough, he said. Now he was questioning if there were any warning signs that he could have missed. He felt that the examination prior to his knee surgery had not been thorough enough. I told him that he would drive himself crazy thinking about that. He stressed adamantly that it was so important to have complete examinations, not just a once over. He said he would keep passing on the importance of this to his friends.

Soon he was up and about more and able to do some work at home. He had listened again to the tape of the last reading from Annmarie. It prompted him to ask her to do another reading, but he wasn't sure yet what he wanted to ask and needed time to think about it. He was interested in information that was coming from the viewpoint of a different consciousness. Annmarie and John would come tomorrow afternoon, and he was looking forward to seeing them. John had worked up a visualization program and taped it for Ray, who was finally ready to try it. We spoke about the forthcoming reading. Ray had first thought he would ask how long he had to live, but then he realized that this was his decision—not that it was being made on a conscious level, but still in his power, his control. No one would be able to tell him with accuracy about that. I agreed completely.

He seemed to be awakening to the knowledge of his own inner spirituality for the first time in his life. It was like a door being unlocked for him. It was exciting and intense. I had always been spontaneous, so in our partnership I was the talker. However, I also had to be careful not to intrude. It would be more wonderful to see him develop and expand day by day and watch him, slowly emerging from his cocoon. He was enjoying himself thoroughly, and I wanted to enjoy it with him.

He was just starting to open his inner doors and had been more expressive in the last few weeks in intimate heart-to-heart communications than in all the years we had been together. Perhaps what Josef said in his reading had been correct. This would be a time for appreciation and growth. Ray was acutely aware and kept expressing to me that it was definitely his choice to live or die, although it was not on a conscious level. He had not denied that he was seriously ill, but he had no intention at that time of leaving. There was a spontaneity about him that I had never seen before. The frequent censoring of his thoughts had ceased. It seemed as if a huge log had broken free of the jam.

Annmarie gave him his reading the next afternoon. It took the form of an intense summation of a large part of his life. It was presented to him that this was his life and that whatever he chose to do was permissible. Josef also told him what problems had arisen from his relationship with his parents and how it related to his present life. I was shocked at the accuracy of the reading, as was Ray. For me, it was the first time that I was able to put the missing pieces of our marriage together. I finally understood why Ray was the way he was. The problems nearly all derived from the hidden rage he carried within himself from life in his father's house.

Later in the reading, Ray asked if he had known Dr. Thomas in a former life. This surprised me because he asked it with such conviction. He had always listened to me talk about reincarnation, but never commented on the subject. He asked Josef this because he was astonished at the close relationship he'd established with Dr. Thomas. He realized that in this type of situation, a close relationship with one's doctor could be formed very quickly, but Ray felt it was more than that. He generally didn't establish this kind of comfort easily or as rapidly as he had done with Dr. Thomas. More than once, he said he felt as if they were old friends.

Josef told him that they had been in the Civil War together. Further, he said that the doctor had fallen off his horse and broken his neck. Ray sat with him and held him while he died, and the doctor had never forgotten his kindness. He wasn't surprised at the explanation nor did he question it.

Ray felt that most of the information rendered by Josef was extremely accurate, so he decided to use it to become more aware and free within himself. This reading brought conscious awareness to him and helped him put his overall situation into some kind of spiritual perspective. John made him an audiotape of a visualization exercise relating to fine-tuning an automobile, and Ray started on his first tape.

A short time later, I myself received a reading from Annmarie. Of course, I asked about Ray and received a lot of support. Josef confirmed that Ray had not given up by any means, but he warned me that he would be "very, very sick" at times. As Ray's system weakened, he would have trouble ridding himself of the toxins. He also warned me to keep him away from any foods that contained nitrates, BHA, BHT, and MSG.

I dreaded having to deal with Ray's diet situation, so I was glad he had at least heard Josef himself. My concern was that the food additives, when combined with the chemo drug, would overload his system. I had been most careful to locate foods with no additives. Ray had had terrible eating habits as a child. He lived on candy and sweets, rarely ate vegetables, and his family members were all voracious meat eaters—as Ray continued to be until he got sick. I was strictly against so much red meat, and he got angry with my preaching. I had been raised differently, as my mother used only fresh vegetables and fruit. During the winter months, she supplemented our diets with what she had preserved. We weren't big on red meat, and sweets were reserved for holidays. I raised my children the same way. I felt it was especially important for girls to eat properly, as the foundation for healthy child-bearing is established in their younger years.

My biggest concern was the amount of red meat he had eaten all his life. I personally felt it was a contributing cause to the cancer. I wondered if I should just let him make the diet decisions himself, though, now that he had the proper information.

I continued to prepare some of the foods suggested, but I couldn't make Ray eat them. It would always be his choice.

CHAPTER FOUR
MY COSMIC DREAM

(February)

By February the emotional impact on the girls of their father's illness was devastating. Up until the time when Ray got sick, Cindy and Gina had shared most of my beliefs on reincarnation, past lives, and the individual being part of the whole. Holly still had many questions, but believed that reincarnation was the only answer to many of life's inequities. Betsy didn't have much to say, but always listened intently during our discussions. However, now their beliefs were being tested, and angry human emotions were emerging. They didn't want to discuss their father's illness in the light of spirituality then, which I realized was a normal reaction. After a few weeks, however, each, in her own way, came to the conclusion that her father's illness was for some higher purpose. My daughters' problem was soon the same as mine. Was it possible to merge inner spiritual truths with raw human emotions? Only time would give us that answer.

None of us knew where Ray's illness would lead us. We were now only two weeks into this nightmare. No one was able to convert their feelings into words. Our feelings changed every day, being yanked back and forth between rage and grief, depression and despair, as well as feeling an utter lack of control over our lives.

On the first of February, two weeks after Ray got sick, spirit blessed me with a magnificent dream. I wanted desperately to stay in my dream because it was such a glorious and emotionally overpowering experience. To put it into words will be almost impossible, but I want to try to share it with you. This conscious encounter with spirit would be my "amazing grace," as I called it, never to be forgotten. It has been a vivid reference point ever since.

I dreamed that I was in an expansive place and that I was expansive with it, yet singular. I was encompassing, yet encompassed by all of it, but still strongly myself. Multitudes of souls were there—thousands of entities like myself who belonged there and were also in spirit. I couldn't see them, but I knew they were present. We were all one, yet each of us was separate. We were in a paradise of complete warmth, happiness, and comfort. I knew that I belonged there and had always belonged there. I saw soft yellow, orange, and white diffused light. I sensed space, lightness, and serenity. I felt tremendous love, freedom, and a strong sense of self; apart and yet together, individual and yet total, all at once. An overpowering feeling of security and peace pervaded this expansiveness. There was no sense of fear, worry, or the slightest anxiety.

I had an overwhelming knowing that I had *always* belonged there, and then I knew that *that* was the real world that, incredibly, I had forgotten. I saw myself glancing back at Earth and yet looking at myself with sadness to realize I could only briefly return there each night. Now a tiny piece of me, only a small part, was slipping back to Earth. I saw myself going down a long tunnel, and I watched as I slipped into my body—feeling a great aversion in having to do so, like drowning or suffocating. I watched in amazement, apart and yet together with my body, finding it all emotionally painful. The Earth felt extremely dense, heavy, and primitive; I was only an infant on Earth compared to what I was in that other realm where I had total power and knowledge, as I had *always* had. I knew that the Earth was not my real home.

I was dumbfounded that we didn't remember all this. The most important discovery was that we spend only a tiny fraction of time in the physical world. I had been so sure that I existed in the physical, spending only brief nights in the astral-spiritual realm, but I had the picture reversed. I was shown in this experience that the physical is actually what we consider the dream state and that it is all a matter of focus.

I also realized how time-oriented and primitive the Earth is compared to the higher realm I was being shown. I experienced "no time"—past, present, or future. All experience just *is*. I felt tremendous joy when I realized my connection with God and my spiritual power. The feeling is not that of power as we know it, but of joy; overwhelming, incomprehensible joy, that's well beyond explaining in earthly terms.

Another awareness affected me strongly. From my lofty vantage point, ongoing earthly problems seemed insignificant when related to the overall scheme of the universe. I could not imagine why I had been so concerned with earth matters, because, in this light, they seemed so trivial. Realizing this made me feel blessedly detached from earth, because I knew now that it wasn't my real home.

In the dream, I was aware of how difficult it would be to connect from there with persons still on Earth because the vibrations are so different. From that realm, one just wasn't interested; a very special spirit was needed to have the will to make the connection. I was aware that the concept of time went hand in hand with the physical dimension, to put some kind of limit on our earthly assignments.

As I was leaving the dream, in that period right before I awakened, I understood fully that only a minute part of our essence could be incorporated into a physical body because the total spirit cannot be contained in such a primitive vessel.

It cannot be contained in anything but total spirit; it is too expansive, too powerful to be fully held in the physical. We *must* forget conscious awareness of the other place during our physical state, in order to be free to work in the physical world, otherwise we would not want to stay on Earth. To experience one's connection with God and the vastness between body and spirit is to know total joy.

Once I was awake it was frustrating to know that I would be unable to share my experience accurately. I felt totally out of sync with my surroundings. I wanted to stay in that beautiful place, but I knew that was impossible. It was not my time to return home to the heavenly realm I had just seen so clearly. Death had been wandering in and out of my thoughts for the past few weeks, and I wondered constantly about it. Now I knew, without a shred of doubt, where my home really was and what would be waiting for me when my time came. Spirit had shown me my real home. I felt that it would be a long time in earth terms before I would return, and that made me sad. I felt a tugging in my mind that this dream had been given to me for Ray's benefit, too. This wondrous experience would not only sustain me through Ray's long illness, but it would abide with me for the rest of my life.

Around the time of my dream, I decided to send it along with my snake dream to Everett Irion at the A.R.E. Mr. Irion is an expert in dream interpretation as well as a scholar on the Revelation of St. John. I needed to know more about my dreams from a spiritual perspective and wanted to make the connection with someone who could give me fresh insight from that point of view. Most times I could grasp a psychological meaning from them, but the dreams I was having during the time of Ray's illness were vastly different, so I wanted someone else's opinion. I knew my dream of February 1 had helped me to remember my real home and my spiritual relationship with the cosmos, but I wanted to hear an expert's opinion.

I told Ray about my wonderful dream. He listened attentively, but didn't offer any comments. In one way it was touchy talking about it with him, since I thought it would make him feel that I was suggesting he was going to die. All I wanted to do was share with him that this is what awaits us all. I didn't speak of the dream to him again until much later.

February expressed herself in snow, dampness, and general bleakness that year. She kept us indoors most of the time but eventually relented, allowing a few days of sunshine when we ventured out into the unaccustomed brightness.

During breaks in the weather, we kept the next scheduled doctor's appointment. The exam was quick. The surgeon was pleased to see that Ray's stomach size had shrunk—a good eight inches. The decrease in bloating most likely was a sign that the chemo was working, drying up the gel-like secretion which carried and spread the cancer cells. Ray had been trying to lose some weight this past year before his surgery. When he noticed the twenty-five-pound weight loss, he remarked dryly, "Not that this is any way to lose weight." His 5'11" well-proportioned frame carried a more suitable weight as a result of the loss. Now we hoped it would remain constant.

Next the doctor drew blood for testing the red-cell count. They didn't like to administer the chemotherapy drugs if the count was too low, because the drug affected the bone marrow which manufactured the red blood cells. To combat this effect, a medication was given along with the chemo drug, aptly nicknamed "rescue pills."

"I'll call you with the results," Dr. Thomas said, and we left.

A few days later Ray was feeling better. Although it had been only three weeks since the surgery, he insisted on driving to a business meeting two hours away. I was concerned, not only that it would be too much for him, but that the weather would turn bad. He told me that he certainly knew what he was capable of doing and what he was not; also, the surgeon had given his approval. I was still edgy and insecure. It led to an argument from which I backed down. The surgery and illness had been so overwhelming to me, I was afraid to get too far away from the hospital and the house. I wondered if my concerns were justified and realized then how frightened I had become of many things—not my normal way of functioning.

We started out, regardless of my reservations. Halfway there the snow moved in, making driving horrendous. It brought stress upon stress, and we were happy to finally arrive at our destination. Ray made his business call and we left. Faced with the slippery ride back home, I was accompanied by my terrific anxiety over the icy roads, my anger at myself for coming, and resentment at him for insisting on taking the trip. I didn't know where my decision boundaries were or if I trusted his. I felt that he wasn't capable of being my protector any more, and I didn't feel comfortable being with him in unfamiliar surroundings. The sickness had changed our relationship in more ways than I realized. However, Ray's spirits had been lifted by his ability to perform his work.

The doctor called soon after with the blood test results, which were good, and the chemo was scheduled for the next day. This time it would be a two-parter: putting in the drug through the abdominal tube, keeping it in overnight, and then draining it off the next day.

The following morning we arrived at the hospital early. Ray liked to have the treatment done first thing, then he had the remainder of the day to rest. I was concerned and anxious about his coming home with the drug still in him.

"Can anything happen?" I asked the doctor.

This was such serious stuff in my mind. Even though I realized the chemotherapy was needed, I never liked it. I knew they were putting severely destructive drugs into him, and I questioned how much and how seriously the rest of his body was suffering from it. The whole idea frightened me terribly. Now I had to bring him home full of the stuff. I didn't have medical experience and wouldn't be able to help him if anything went wrong.

Dr. Thomas assured me that it would be fine through the night, but I was still on edge. He remarked to Ray, "I'm impressed," when he saw how much the stomach swelling had decreased. He admitted that he hadn't expected such quick results and was pleased with the progress. The medication was stronger this time, so Ray was tired when the treatment was finished. We left the hospital, and the chemo drug—still in—came home with us. I assured myself that Betsy was only a phone call away, as was the doctor and an ambulance, and Gina was in the house, too. However, things went well that night; there were no problems, and he went back the next day to have the drug removed.

Ray tried the visualization tape that John had made for him, associating his body with the tuning of an automobile. However, Ray said he couldn't follow someone else's voice guiding him through the suggested visualization. "I'm going to try it myself," he told me.

I really shouldn't have been surprised, knowing his creativity in everything he did, so I asked him, "How are you going to do that?"

"By letting my mind run free," he answered.

I knew he had read some of the books I had bought. He had been reading Simonton's *Getting Well Again*, and I had also given him *Edgar Cayce on ESP*, by Doris Agee. The books contained several different approaches to visualization, so, after a day or so, I asked him what he had come up with.

"As soon as I wake up, around 5:15 a.m., I lay very still and quiet for awhile, trying to relax," he said. Then he told me he picked a definite spot on the ceiling and concentrated only on that spot. Then, he let his mind "run loose." He tried to direct his consciousness down to his lower body cavity and go inside, visualizing what was happening in there. I was surprised that he had such a good grip on it and asked him how he had come about doing it that way.

He explained that he combined all that he had been reading, along with his own feelings; in fact, he'd already been doing it for several days. That morning it had been hard going. He said that he "drifted" like he had done in the out-of-body experience in the hospital. Then he described his vivid, remarkable experience in detail, which I later wrote down.

He had found himself standing on a tiny ten-by-twenty foot island, surrounded by fast-flowing, clear water. The island was a bare piece of dark brown earth. It seemed as though he knew exactly where he was. He was calm and relaxed. The island was in a large dark cavern. As he looked around, out to the left side and front there was a huge dark cliff; to the right side were many entrances into the cavern, through which water was entering. He was in the center point for all the flowing water.

Someone was standing on the forward part of the island. It was a man, but Ray couldn't see who it was. He walked over to the person and was surprised to discover Dr. Thomas. He was wearing a gray suit, red tie, and golashes on his feet. Ray was wearing his brown pants, brown sweater, and no boots. Dr. Thomas started to point to the cliffs of the cavern to the left of the island, then said, "See that whole section in the front? It's all cleared up. We must work on the rear section now."

As Ray looked to the other side of the cavern in the rear and right front where the water was flowing in, he noticed many small (golf-ball size) reddish-purple growths on the cavern walls. As the two men looked at them, Dr. Thomas said, "They're next. We must work on them next."

On the right and rear two sides were violent reactions between the clear water (medicine) and the growths, similar to boiling water and steam. The growths were being defeated because Dr. Thomas was counting them as they vanished. The whole area was dark, but wherever the two looked, a bright white spotlight came down from the top of the cavern and lit it.

Dr. Thomas waded into the water to check the clarity of it. He had a rubber glove on his right hand and scooped up the water. Then he said, "See the water from both sides of the island? It's going to your kidneys, and they're throwing out all the growths."

Ray saw the waters being emptied into one large cavity. He knew his kidneys were down that large dark hole.

"At that point I came into full awareness and found the whole experience calming and relaxing," he said, adding, "What do you think of that?"

I stared at him. "You saw all that?" I asked. We discussed the remarkable symbols of illness he'd seen during his apparently self-induced visualization. I was truly astonished at his facility. He interpreted the water as the chemo drug and the reddish-purple growths as the tumors. When I asked him what the spotlight was he said, matter of factly, "I think it was God."

He had told me that he would try visualizing by himself when he was ready. He finally did, and what wonderful results he achieved!

We were excited about Ray's visualization and discussed sharing it with the doctor. I wondered if there could be any medical merit to it. After all, he had seen his insides with as much detail as the surgeon had—if not more. But Ray decided against telling him. I didn't have much to say in the decision. It was his experience, and the spiritual pilgrim hiding within the engineer was not yet ready to reveal himself. Ultimately the whole family agreed that telling the doctor would be a bad idea.

I felt that Ray's entry inside his body had been more than a simple visualization process. He had initially visualized it, but then the energy took hold and seemed to carry him away on its own momentum. Ray felt that it had given him some kind of a "right of entrance" into a formerly inaccessible region. To anyone who has cancer, lack of control over the disease is devastating, but this experience had given Ray a sense of that missing control.

Ray felt well enough toward the end of February to plan a business trip to his home office outside Boston, so we decided to take the AmTrak sleeper. During our brief stay in Boston, Ray had another unusual "meditation," as he called them, in the motel room.

He seemed to have the uncanny ability to zero in on a subject he wanted to know about and get the needed information. It was some sort of lucid psychic phenomenon that I assumed was coming from his spirit, but I couldn't put a label on it. He was very matter of fact about the event and didn't ask too many questions. He just accepted it and thought it was interesting. I wondered why he had not asked to see a cure or asked for help in becoming involved in a more physical way with his healing.

For this particular "meditation" he awakened at 5:15 a.m. as usual, found a focal point on the ceiling, and started to visualize. Soon, as before, he was able to mentally enter his body, but this time found himself on the island alone. Yet it looked exactly the same as when he was there before. Someone, whom he could not see but heard silently, told him to give names to the areas which he and Dr. Thomas had identified in his earlier island meditation. It seemed important to do so.

The first area he named was where he had seen the turmoil and battling. He called that part St. Joan's Fire—a combination of St. Elmo's Fire, for the energy being expended in that area, and Joan, his chemotherapy nurse who administered the drug. Then he looked at the right bottom area, the original cancer site, which was the worst area where much had to be done. He could see a lot of red-purplish hanging growths. He named this section Rosemary's Alley—a play on the movie title *Rosemary's Baby*, for the devastation involved in that area. Farther up from there and toward the back was the third area where more growths also were present. However, this part required less work, and he named it Andy's Mountain because it was higher up than the other two areas. Andy had been an old friend, who years before had beaten cancer. There were no spotlights this time, but there was enough light to see everything. The area that was cleared up he didn't name.

Ray's meditations made us curious to know if they would reveal further insight into what was happening or was about to happen in his body. We left Boston that afternoon on the long train ride home and were happy to be back in our own bed that night.

The following morning Ray received another message. He told me that he couldn't accept that it had been a dream. He knew it happened, because he thought he was conscious as it unfolded. It was an encounter with my deceased mother, Jessie.

Ray and Jessie had always had an unusual relationship. Most of the time, he was more patient with her than I was. She had been a difficult, childlike person, very critical of him as she was with most people. As she grew older, their relationship changed and she became very fond of him.

I watched Ray closely and asked him to tell me in detail what had happened. He told me that he had found himself sitting in the den in his blue p.j.'s, robe, and slippers. He was about to read the *Intelligencer* newspaper he had picked up. He had just come down from upstairs after reading the *Inquirer*. It was in the afternoon. As he was sitting in his beige lounge chair, Jessie came around from behind the chair. He assumed she had been in the bathroom and was on her way out. It never crossed his mind that she was dead. It was all very matter of fact, he said. She had on a white blouse and a gray-and-black plaid taffeta skirt and looked good—like she did twenty-five years ago, with a bounce in her step. "Hi, Jess," Ray called out.

She stopped by his chair, looked right at him, and said, "Hi, Ray. How are you feeling?"

He answered, "Much better."

"I understand you had a little bout. (This was a favorite word my mother always used to denote any kind of difficulty). Don't worry about it. In a year you'll be all cleared up." Then she said, "O.K., I'll be in touch," and walked off into the kitchen. He thought I was in the kitchen and that she was going through the door to see me.

Ray continued, "I sat up in bed with a start. I want to tell you I have never had such a dream before. It was unbelievable!"

I couldn't distinguish if it were a vision, an out-of-body experience, a particularly lucid dream, or some type of time interruption. I detected some clues when he mentioned the *Intelligencer* and *Inquirer* newspapers. He was looking for news, so when he came downstairs his inquiry was not on the intellectual level. My mother asked him about his health and then belittled the cancer by calling it "a little bout." She told him he would be "cleared up" in about a year. Right away Ray interpreted this as a positive message from my mother. It was a positive spiritual encounter, but when I thought about it, I wasn't sure if my mother was referring to his illness being cleared up on a physical level or if it indicated more of a spiritual lesson. We would only know in time what this visit truly meant. I was astonished at Ray's psychic ability to connect with her in such a vivid way.

The names he had associated with in his island meditation—Andy, Rosemary's Baby, St. Elmo's Fire, along with the visit from my mother—all had settings of twenty-five years ago. He wondered about the significance of that particular time period in his life. He didn't have any answers that morning, but he felt it was all beneficial information and hoped it would continue. Over the next week he had numerous paranormal experiences during his meditations. With each of these, he returned free of pain. On his first visit to the island, he noticed that he had an hour or so of relief, but each meditation after that relieved him for a slightly longer time.

I asked him how he had felt in the hospital after his first out-of-body episode as far as pain was concerned. He told me that it had been the first time he felt pain free.

Ray said how much he looked forward to talking about these events. It was the highlight of his day when we could intimately discuss these new experiences. They offered a two-fold blessing: bringing him relief from his pain—even though for only a few hours—and drawing him into closer conversations with me. Later, he would announce, "I've decided to stop my medication during the day."

February continued to bring him many more beautiful occurrences. He went into his meditations holding onto the sensation of how he felt when he had no pain. Doors opened into the deepest parts of his psyche. He couldn't understand where all the information was coming from, but he did know that his meditations were bringing him hours of relief. That was indeed a great gift. He looked forward to connecting with his inner self and always came back relaxed and free from depression. He knew that the visit from my mother, which had affected him strongly, had not been an actual physical meeting, but he could not fathom why it was so difficult to differentiate the visit from waking reality. "How can something that was so real, not be real?" he asked me.

Near the end of February Ray was free of all pain medication. He decided to keep on practicing his meditations, to open himself to all new experiences—no matter how unorthodox they appeared to be.

Lou came by to see us and to join with us in another prayer

communion. Like before, we prayed silently together and called in the light. I had been able to visualize brilliant white light, making it strong and powerful in the room. Our prayer session was intense, and my tears came quickly. Lou surprised me by starting a steady chanting, which took on a monotonic, humming quality. I had never heard this before and felt myself aligning and attuning to it. He was calling to God in this steady, rhythmic chant, and I felt carried along and engulfed by its sweet wave, instinctively joining in. As the steady cadence swept over and through me, it seemed to vibrate from all directions. Beautiful colors appeared in my mind's eye: first softly pale, then strong shades of green, purple, and red. I was emotionally overcome and wept quietly, sensing a feeling of lightness in my body akin to lifting. I experienced a strong presence of spirit in the room. I calmed myself and looked at Ray. He was completely relaxed in the chair, his face mirroring peaceful tranquillity.

Lou swept his hands over Ray about three inches above his body, clearing his aura. He told him that he must forgive himself. The light evidently conveyed insight to Lou about what Ray was feeling. I was astounded that he had received this information, because Ray and I both knew it was something he needed to do. Ray was hard on himself; he'd had a problem with guilt over the loss of his job, his present inability to perform in his new job, and the general guilt he had carried with him from childhood. Obviously, it continued into the time of his illness. Lou told him that his aura had changed greatly since he first visited him in the hospital. He noticed that his physical body had changed, too. We were all elated.

Ray announced happily that he had a tingling on the soles of his feet and that he was totally relaxed, calm, and without physical discomfort. That day I felt deeply connected with our great loving God, and I was overwhelmed with joy. It had been an uplifting and spiritual evening.

Ray had had a CAT scan done, and we were waiting for the

results. With all the visualization work, we were anxious for good news. A new cough had started up a few days before and was now becoming persistent, irritating his stomach and making him uncomfortable. He couldn't meditate because of the constant coughing. I called the doctor, who prescribed a different medication to break the cycle. The doctor advised us that he would be sending a visiting nurse more often to monitor Ray's lungs. He didn't want to run into any trouble. Ray felt much better in the evening after taking the new medication and wanted to take Gina and me out to dinner. I thought he should rest, but it was easier to go along with him. Again he assured me that he knew what he was capable of doing, so we went. Dinner out was a treat. We enjoyed the atmosphere of the softly lit dining room and our meal. Gina remarked what great spirits he was in; she felt uplifted by his exhuberance.

February dealt us one last stunning blow. Ray got up that day with a sharp, stabbing pain in both sides of his back. He was hoarse and wheezy. I called the doctor, who told me to bring him to the emergency room immediately. After we arrived at the hospital, x-rays revealed pneumonia in both lungs and pleurisy. The doctor also noticed that his stomach was bloated, and it concerned him greatly. This had developed practically overnight, even though the visiting nurse had been checking his lungs every other day.

We couldn't understand how this happened, since he had been monitored so carefully. The doctor prescribed a strong antibiotic and suggested he stay overnight in the hospital. But Ray was adamant about going home, so the doctor instructed him that as long as he could take medication by mouth, he could leave. However, in forty-eight hours, if he were no better, the doctor would have to readmit him to the hospital.

I called the girls from the hospital. They, too, questioned how this could happen. I suggested that maybe he had been doing too much. The germ had done its foul deed despite our constant vigilance. The girls wanted him to stay in the hospital overnight, but I knew how desperately he wanted to come home. So, I assured myself that Betsy was within calling distance, and Gina was with us should an emergency arise. As soon as we left, however, my apprehension turned to nervous nausea.

Later, at home, Ray managed to drink lots of fluid and got some sherbet down. He was so down and depressed over the terrible diagnosis. All the progress he had accomplished after the surgery seemed unimportant to him then, though I kept reminding him that this was just a temporary setback. Gina sat with him for awhile, and he fell asleep. During the night his fever broke, and I felt a little bit better.

The next day Dr. Thomas called with the CAT scan results, but he really couldn't tell us much. He said that he wanted to use it as a baseline to measure how well the chemo was working relative to shrinking the tumors. I wished they had gone ahead and done the scan when it was mentioned back in January. I was now angry that they hadn't taken it then, knowing they could be using it now as a better baseline. Dr. Thomas's only input had been what the surgeon observed visually during the surgery. Until now, he had nothing on which to base Ray's progress or lack of it.

Ray's forty-eight hours were nearly up, and we hadn't seen much improvement. He had not gotten any worse, nor had there been any positive improvement. I called in the progress report to the doctor, remarking over the phone that maybe Ray had been doing too much. He exploded in anger at me. He was loaded with rage over the turn of events, and I guess I was a convenient target. I was always looking for the reasons that could cause such severe physical ups and downs; and maybe there just weren't any.

Sadly, Dr. Thomas determined that there had been no definite improvement. He ordered Ray back into the hospital. The medical team felt there was an obstruction or infection in the colon because of the fresh swelling that was adding to his other miseries. At least, his lungs were more clear after taking the strong antibiotic. A vivid image came into my mind as I remembered Ray diving into a pool and swimming the entire length of it under water. Our granddaughter Sarah stood at the other end watching him. She had gotten worried when her "Pop-Pop" had been under so long and asked me how he could hold his breath that long. That had been only a year before.

Dr. Thomas took a sample of fluid from the stomach tube and walked it over to the lab to see what was going on. Later that day he came back with the results. The culture, he said, didn't show any surprises. It appeared that bacteria from the colon had gotten into the abdomen, causing peritonitis and swelling. They continued to culture this bacteria. I panicked at the diagnosis of peritonitis, because I knew how deadly serious it was. Peritonitis is a general infection of the abdomen, which is life threatening in itself. My God, what more could happen to him? He was in such a serious state, and they tossed these terrible diagnostic terms about like he had nothing more than a common cold.

The surgeon ordered three different broad spectrum antibiotics. He was also considering taking the stomach catheter tube out but then decided against that because it was still doing its job. The anemia was back, too, contributing to his overall distress; transfusions were started. They had decided surgery was not necessary; long treatment with antibiotics should remedy the situation. He was given an inhalator to loosen lung congestion, and finally in a day or two we saw improvement.

Dr. Thomas was sure the broad spectrum of antibiotics would be on target. Remarkably, Ray's fever was coming down, the red count was going up, and his lungs were clearing. He was eating and felt much better physically, but he was so depressed emotionally about his perceived loss of ground.

I was still stunned from the vicious blow and full of despair—right back where I started. Going over the events of those last few weeks confused me even more. The medical evidence had said he was progressing well, and Ray had been doing better physically. Even Lou had perceived the beginnings of his healing.

How many of these uncontrollable catastrophes could Ray withstand? What would happen in the next two days or the two days after that? If the spirit of God was entering and helping, why was this happening? I was extremely tentative about permitting positive feelings back in, even though the doctors were telling me that he was coming along. I didn't know if I could take another disappointment. The changes in his condition were so rapid; I felt as if I were following a bouncing ball.

Ray would be able to come home in a day or two, but I couldn't even think about that. I was frightened and wanted him to stay where he was. I felt that I couldn't take care of him, while the hospital offered security. I was really surprised that I felt so strongly about it. I wouldn't mention this to Ray; all he could think about was coming home.

The girls had been so helpful and supportive. Having Gina with me was wonderful. Holly was back and forth constantly, and Cindy and Betsy stopped by after work. I had to remember how fortunate I was in having all their support and love.

More days were behind us, and Ray continued to improve. Dr. Thomas told us that the culture results had finally isolated the bacteria in the intestines, which he called a "a nasty bastard" of a germ. "But," he said, "now that I know what suit it wears, I can get it."

The doctors tried to figure out how the bug got from the intestines into the abdomen. Dr. Thomas first thought it had perforated the original cancer site and gone into the abdomen, but this didn't show on the CAT scan. Then it was suggested the germ was from dead cancer cells being sloughed off from the tumors. More x-rays would be taken to determine how this germ got into the abdomen. His lungs were clearing up nicely; he called the lung inhalator his "peace pipe."

The following Monday morning when I walked into Ray's room I caught him dozing. He was dreaming and his lips were moving. Although I was very quiet, he sensed my presence and opened his eyes. He smiled at me, and I knew he had been back on his island. After I hugged and kissed him, he proceeded to tell me about it.

Both Dr. Thomas and he were in a boat, a small gray, shallow, wooden rowboat, using poles so they could maneuver the boat. They both had on black slickers and hats, like fishermen. The water was coming down off the walls. Some water was clear and some was reddish purple. It was raining into the water. They were up Rosemary's Alley, the area inside his abdomen which he had previously seen and which needed the most work. In reality it was the most sensitive place in his stomach, presenting him with the most problems. (He told me he had pain when he woke up and felt it was from going into the alley to check.) He continued on and told me, when they were up Rosemary's Alley, that Dr. Thomas said to him, "Don't worry. I can steer the treatments into this area only. I can give it a good barrage because we haven't made much progress in here." I also hoped he could barrage it in Ray's waking life.

Ray remarked that it seemed as if he and the doctor were busy when they were in there and the tumors were shrinking some. But the infection was the culprit now. He thought that the rain coming down was the infection from the germ. I thought the vision was exciting, but I wanted to wait and see what the doctor had to say about that area named Rosemary's Alley. Ray felt excited that he was able to get back again inside his abdomen, and his depression quickly lifted. February finally exited, and March entered like the roar of a lion.

CHAPTER FIVE

RESURRECTION

(March)

By the beginning of March, the physical ups and downs of Ray's illness had overwhelmed us all. We had faced sickness before, as well as some other emotionally taxing events over the years with the kids, but nothing as tragic as this.

Ray and I sat talking in his room on the Monday morning Dr. Thomas was to release him from the hospital. He was feeling better and trying to put the last horrendous week of pleurisy and pneumonia into some kind of perspective. "I can't wait to get home so I can start my meditations again," he said.

Meditating had become vitally important to him. He benefited immensely from the results which actually brought him freedom from pain, a deep relaxation, and a lifting of his depression. I leaned back and let out a long breath of relief. I was elated to see him beginning to look ahead again. He was more at peace that morning and felt that the antibiotics would do their job. I was beginning to sense a faint stirring of hope revive within me and it felt good.

We were discussing our plans for the days ahead when Dr. Thomas walked into the room. He chatted with us for awhile, then said he wanted to check the abdominal catheter. He reached across Ray and removed the catheter cap. To our shock, the tube blew like a small volcano, spewing with great force a dark discharge, accompanied by a terrible odor. "What's wrong?" I asked, getting up quickly. Visibly upset, the doctor ordered immediate x-rays. Within minutes Ray was being placed on a gurney.

The situation had changed so rapidly that I just stood there unable to comprehend what was happening. Then, a sense of detachment seemed to overtake me. I felt myself becoming a distant observer again, just looking on. I fought the feeling, not believing how outwardly calm I was. They wheeled Ray out the door to radiology and left me standing alone in his empty room. I was stunned, but I knew I had to move. Instantly, I was out the door and running down the hall after Ray. The two technicians on either side of the gurney told me over their shoulders that Ray wouldn't be back in his room for at least an hour and a half.

I knew I had to get out of there. So I got myself onto the elevator and headed for the front exit. Consciously, I decided to put it out of my mind, just pretend it wasn't happening. I had to have time to decide how I was going to survive this latest onslaught. I told myself that I would come back in an hour or so and that everything would be all right. I reminded myself not to panic and decided not to call the girls until I had more information. But where could I go? Suddenly, a vision of the fabric store down the highway popped into my mind.

I would stop there and browse and not think about anything. I wandered around the store for awhile, picking things up absently until the anxiety worked its way through my defense system. Then I knew that I just had to be with someone. I hoped Betsy was home, but I couldn't remember her work schedule that week. I didn't bother calling her. I just pointed the car toward her house and drove. She opened the door, took one look at my face, and asked, "What's the matter? What's happened?"

I took a deep breath and stood mute for a long moment before I was finally able to tell her what was going on. Betsy just stared at me, giving her nurse's mind time to evaluate the frightening situation.

"He'll be all right," she said. "Maybe the cap coming off the tube will allow for more drainage. They know what they're doing, Mom." I guess she didn't know what else to say to me. She asked what time the x-rays would be finished, and I told her around 4:30 or 5:00 p.m. and that I'd call the hospital then.

"I'll make some coffee," she said. "Just sit down and calm yourself. Everything will be all right." I prayed that she was right.

At 4:30 p.m. I dialed Ray's room. "Where are you?" he demanded, and I knew by his tone that he was angry.

"They told me you wouldn't be back for at least an hour and a half," I said. "What's happened?" I could feel my stomach churn. I knew that something was very wrong.

"They're pretty sure I'm going to need surgery," he said. "You better get back here right away."

I told Betsy and asked her to have her sisters come to the hospital as soon as they could. Then I dashed out the door. I felt panic hit me so hard that I had to sit for a minute in the car to collect myself. I couldn't deny that I wanted to run away. My first reaction was fear that he wouldn't survive another surgery. Then, I truly didn't know how I was going to get through it this time. The fact that I had no choice only added another level of anxiety. That was one of the most difficult facets I encountered throughout his illness: losing my power to make choices.

I knew the consequences would be serious when I saw the tube erupt. I hadn't been able to face the ramifications of it when I left the hospital, but now another surgery was flying right at me. I had to deal with it, like it or not. My overwhelming concern for Ray was unbearable. It had only been six weeks since his last major operation, and he'd just gotten over pneumonia and pleurisy.

These thoughts poured through my mind as I raced back to the hospital and up to his floor. I entered near the nurse's station and saw the surgeon at the desk, phone in hand. He looked up at me as I hurried through the door. "I was trying to phone you," he said. "We've scheduled Ray for surgery."

I looked up at the clock and saw that it was a little past 5:00 p.m. and, incredibly, he told me that Ray would be going into the operating room within the hour. Barking orders at the nurses, he put his pen down on the desk and walked over to me. I was treading water in a sea of routine hospital commotion, but his approach had thrust me back into the bustle of reality. I knew it was extremely serious as I listened to the orders being given to the staff to prepare for Ray's surgery. There was an urgency to it that frightened me terribly.

The surgeon explained they had completed both barium and dye tests and were sure that the cancer at the original site had perforated the colon and leaked into the abdominal cavity, allowing matter from the intestines to enter there. That was what had caused the eruption from the tube. It had been the root cause of the infection. Ray would need a colostomy to stop the leakage into the abdominal cavity—it was a life-threatening situation. The infection from the perforation had spread extensively, and no amount of antibiotic would stop it. They wouldn't let me see Ray until the nurse finished prepping him for surgery.

The girls arrived one by one. We huddled together in silence. "He's not going to make it, Mom," Holly wept softly.

"He's strong," Betsy said, but her voice quivered. "They have to go in and fix it."

Cindy got up and paced the hall, while Gina sat quietly with me. I wanted it to be over—not just this surgery, but the whole event. I kept thinking how cruel this was. Either I wanted him well or I wanted it over. Why prolong it if he wasn't going to get better? I couldn't stand it. I couldn't stand to see him suffering so.

Finally, the nurse was finished and we went in. Ray knew that he had no choice and was terribly upset. He would have to undergo major surgery again. His face was so pale and grave. I tried to comfort him, but he told me, "Don't worry. I'm not going anywhere. I'll see you later." Yet I heard the fear in his voice. Then they came in and put him on another gurney. We gathered closely together and walked down the hall beside him as they rolled the gurney toward the operating room for the second time.

None of us was sure if his poor sick body would be able to withstand more trauma. I told myself that this would be the last time. Why wasn't there a choice, I screamed inwardly to myself. We didn't want him to die, but the surgeon said he would die if this wasn't done. It was becoming clear to us how little modern medicine can accomplish in situations like this. The doctors were competent, the drugs reflected the latest technology, and research had come a long way. Yet here was my husband, despite his courageous fight, facing more surgery.

Awful thoughts of him not coming back were running through my head as we walked alongside him, talking softly, not wanting to release him into the forbidding area of the O.R. The doors yawned open, they pushed him through, then the doors rapidly swung shut. We were left standing before a vacant space, his image hanging in the emptiness. He was now in the hands of those caretakers in the sterile masks and white shoes. I wanted to scream at everyone—even at God for allowing this in His universe.

I felt totally alone even in the midst of my own family. I had to blame someone, because I didn't want to blame Ray for taking this journey. I knew he wasn't doing it consciously, but my emotional side was being irrational. My inner self still knew what was going on, but my outer self screamed in rage at the universe. I was here and not with God, and that made me human. I felt I had the right to rant and rave and shake my fists at the heavens.

We stood in the empty hallway, looking at the closed doors, then we shuffled down the corridor, spaced out and separate, to the waiting room. We would be there two-and-a-half hours. There was nothing that would relieve our anxiety. Everyone was up and down, back and forth to the coffee shop, just for something to do. We also visited the chapel and asked for God's help. At that point I felt dead inside and doubted if my prayers would even be heard. There wasn't anything to say to each other either. Each was lost in her own thoughts, wondering how Ray would be able to survive.

We waited for what seemed an intolerable amount of time when Cindy suddenly spotted the surgeon coming out of the O.R. We gathered near the door and waited for him to come in. He told us immediately that all had gone extremely well, under the circumstances. They had found no new surprises, except the impression that there had actually been some shrinkage of the tumors overall.

The surgeon hadn't wanted to explore any more than was necessary. He had cut a small piece out of the colon, then taken each end and hooked it up to a bag on the outside of the abdomen. There was a possibility that it could be put back together at some later date—at least there was that hopeful option. They were pleased that the infection in the abdomen had walled itself off. They had put more drainage tubes into that area to draw off the infection. Transfusions would be continued to keep ahead of the repercussions from the surgery. The surgeon said that the lower colon was healthy and that the small intestines were not affected. This, he said, was a surprising bonus.

We were so relieved that Ray had come through the surgery alive that all of us loudly thanked God. I honestly hadn't known if he would have the strength to make it; that was my main concern. I thanked God again that it was over and that all had gone well. The doctor remarked that Ray was talking to them in the recovery room and that he was amazed at his stamina and overall recoupability.

Then we saw Ray being wheeled down the hall. He looked awful, yet he was talking. His face, though, had a sickly pallor and he was in terrible pain. I was furious that the universe would allow this kind of journey. Inside I lashed out at the world, but not having anything tangible to channel my rage toward only left me more frustrated. I looked down at Ray, wondering what lay ahead for him, then felt guilty because I was worrying about myself, too.

Talking tired him, so they advised us to go home. He was heavily sedated so that he could sleep through the night. We each whispered to him a few minutes, hugged him, and said good-night, then filed silently out of the room. We walked into the starkly lit hall, across the shiny waxed corridors, and into the elevator. I remember that walk so well because I wanted to scream and pound my fists against the walls. We had cried and cried, but the force of the illness was relentless and showed no compassion. Frustration and anger were my constant companions now. I dreaded the coming week because I knew how much trauma Ray would have to fight again. Then, there would be the long recovery ahead.

The next morning, after a sleepless night, I didn't even want to get out of bed. I felt that I needed to stay in my bedroom for the rest of my life and never come out. I wanted to pull the covers up over my head and bolt the door. I was sorely tempted to do it, but then I felt ashamed. If the situation had been reversed, Ray would have been there for me; there was no question in my mind about that. Thoughts of how he must have been feeling that morning came to my mind. So, knowing that physical distance would not solve my dilemma, I threw the covers back and psyched myself to face the day ahead.

When I called to check on Ray, the nurse said that he was out of danger, but that the night had not been good. They had awakened him often to take vital signs. Knocked out by the surgery itself and the long night, he was sleeping late, so we decided to wait until noon to see him. When the girls and I walked into his room, we were surprised to see him sitting up in a chair. Our internist was there examining him and told us that he was doing well. He asked me later if I wanted to see what had been done in surgery because, although Ray would learn to change his bag before he was discharged, I would have to help him with the dressing. I wasn't prepared to do it just then, so I declined.

The doctor ordered more potent shots for the pain and advised us that Ray would be doing a lot of sleeping through the initial recovery. They brought in a blower machine to expand his lungs and get rid of the aftereffects of the anesthetic. Betsy checked the equipment over. I noticed that she did this automatically.

I called later around dinner time to check on him. He wanted us to come back. He was doing much better in the evening. His vital signs were good, and his spirits were somewhat up. Holly did some wisecracking, and he was up to responding back. Cindy told him what was going on at work, and Gina told him that her fiance, Brian, would be coming soon for a visit. The room had a more peaceful feeling to it that night, and Ray was much calmer. Somehow I felt that there was help around him—spiritual help that was supporting him. The feeling comforted me, too.

Time had no other dimension for me than to measure those long, initial days of recovery. Ray continued to improve. However, one of the young surgeons on the team remarked to me that this had been a different and difficult case. The operating surgeon told me two days later that Ray was recuperating much better than expected, and he was pleased. I somehow knew that Ray would stay here for awhile with us. My friends Joanne and Annmarie agreed after they visited him.

Later, Betsy's friend Becky, who was also a nurse there, told her that Ray was the talk of the hospital. The staff hadn't seen anyone bounce back as he had; they were saying that he was a marvelous patient. We relayed this to Ray, and he beamed. I was sure that I couldn't have been as patient and uncomplaining. It was really amazing when I realized the patience he had developed. In many ways, patience had never been his strong suit.

I spoke to Dr. Thomas and mentioned that the surgeon had said the tumors were shrinking. He questioned me on this, because the surgeon was an absolute realist and didn't give an inch of encouragement if he didn't have definite facts. Dr. Thomas, though, was pleased. I wondered why the surgeon had failed to mention this to him. I assumed that he had been too engrossed with the surgical details and simply forgot to pass on the information. However, Dr. Thomas felt there were still serious problems at the original cancer site, and that concerned him. I heard him, but didn't respond.

Ray's progress continued. Three days later the surgeon took one drain tube out of the abdomen. He advised Ray that he would be able to go home as soon as the infection cleared to their satisfaction. Dr. Thomas brought up his concern about the original cancer site again and told me it was still putting out live cancer cells. He reminded me how aggressive this cancer was. He had looked at it under the microscope and wasn't sure how he would pinpoint that particular place with the chemo. Ray smiled at me after Dr. Thomas left. "You know what area that is, don't you?" he said and grinned with satisfaction. I thought for a minute where the original cancer site was located and realized it was in the rear of his lower right abdomen. "That's Rosemary's Alley, isn't it?"

"Exactly," Ray answered with a gleam. "Dr. Thomas told me on the island that he could steer the drug into that area and give it a good barrage. Let's hope he can figure out a way to target it, in this reality. It ought to be interesting."

Incredible, I thought. The areas that Ray and Dr. Thomas had identified in the intitial island meditation hadn't been mere symbols at all. He had seen this area in the meditation and realized, well before the eruption and surgery, that it would be the problem spot. Although I wasn't sure anything could have been done before this, the confirmation of what he had seen in Rosemary's Alley was important to Ray. I hoped he could soon get back again onto his island.

During the following week, Ray felt a little better each day, and friends and acquaintances streamed in and out of his room. Gina's fiance, Brian, arrived from Northern Ireland for a visit. Brian had a cheerful, energetic demeanor about him; he was like a breath of fresh air. He came right to the hospital, and he and Ray had a good visit. Sometimes I thought the visiting was too much for Ray, but he enjoyed it and it diverted his mind from his illness. He was healing nicely. If he continued with his progress, he would be coming home soon.

On the following Tuesday the enterostomal therapist came to Ray's room to speak with me. Her specialty was in colostomies. She showed me what I needed in order to help Ray, if necessary, with the bags and other paraphernalia. I admired her courage in having chosen this field. Ray had already had his lessons with her and was doing well. He confided to me that if this had happened twenty years before, it would have been much more difficult for him to accept the colostomy bag. Because the incision had to heal from the inside out, a great deal of the wound was open. It would eventually close, but its appearance frightened me at first. I kept telling him not to move around too much, but he laughed at me, saying, "It's okay. Really." I thought to myself at that moment, he's not standing on the sidelines observing this time.

We had been waiting for a release date. Later that day, Dr. Thomas told Ray that he could leave the following morning. I felt anxious about his release, but I wanted him home. Doubting my own capabilities in managing a situation was new to me, and it made me uncomfortable. The doctors weren't too concerned when Ray developed a fever after surgery and his white count was up, indicating an infection. They intended to monitor him closely.

For the first time in weeks I received an important dream which I remembered upon awakening. In my dream, I was standing on a dark one-lane road. It was snowing heavily. The snow was muffling all sound and had enclosed me on a piece of earth in a black, desolate place. The whiteness and closeness of the snow made me feel isolated from the rest of the world. I felt encapsulated in my own time and space, in absolute silence.

As I stood there, I knew that two cars were coming from different directions on the one-lane road and that there was only room enough for one car. Neither driver could see the lights of the other. I could feel them coming—dark, hurtling, hidden objects, charged with tremendous energy, speeding through the blackness and the heavy snow on a collision course. It was impossible to warn them. I thought perhaps they would see each other's lights. The knowledge that they would collide right on the spot where I stood caused me such panic that I was frozen to the road. I had to get out of their way. I turned around and saw a large open cornfield behind me.

The dry dead parts of the corn stalks were sticking up like rows of soldiers. As I darted among them, the two cars came streaking by with the energy of a thousand cannon balls. They shot by each other and hurtled down the road. I was astonished and couldn't understand why they had not collided. I looked down the road to the right and saw a large, brilliantly lit intersection. The brightness from the overhead street lights glared down on a man who entered the intersection to cross. As I wondered where the intersection had come from, the car that had passed me from the left streaked through the crossing and struck the man. People ran around excitedly; then an ambulance came. I woke up with a start, not knowing the outcome of the accident. The dream had been frightening. I could still feel the isolation of the place.

Throughout the day, the imagery of the dream never left me, so I knew I could uncover a message in it if I tried. I interpreted the snow as a symbol of the spirit of God. My standing isolated in the dark meant that I was feeling cut off and needed to find that spirit again within myself. I saw the two cars as representing the relationship between Ray and me. We were coming from two different directions and were sure to collide on the narrow road if one of us didn't change his or her path. In the dream, neither driver could see the other's lights. That was our big problem. Most of the time we couldn't see each other's "light." We hadn't been able to communicate intimately and had, therefore, collided in many ways over the years.

Then I realized that I had to move out of the way. I took this as meaning that I needed to move my ego aside and let spirit take over. I knew that the man in the intersection was Ray. It was clear that he had big decisions to make, and I felt strongly that these decisions were on the spiritual level, outside of his personality consciousness. His being hit by the car was his body being invaded by cancer. In life, as in the dream, I didn't know the outcome. I didn't know what his choice had been or even if he'd yet made it.

The dream helped me in several ways. It reinforced my need to get closer to God within myself. It also seemed to promise that if I could manage to keep my ego out of the way, I'd be a lot better off and maybe even of more help to Ray.

Gina, Brian, and I went to bring Ray home from the hospital the next day. We carried everything down to the car and were finally on our way. I thanked God that Betsy was near and that the visiting nurse would be coming frequently. It was a beautiful day. We thought perhaps the shining sun had been arranged for him. I felt, after receiving my last dream, that spirit was definitely guiding us, and I wondered how bumpy the ride ahead was going to be.

A few days later, Gina and Brian were off to Mexico for a week. Ray wanted to drive with me to the airport, and I didn't know what to say. I couldn't believe that he would even consider going. However, before our conversation went any further, he decided that he wasn't up to it. I thanked God that he had made the decision on his own.

That evening Ray's temperature dropped to normal, and he announced that he was hungry. We felt elated. I allowed my positiveness to build. His temperature continued to remain stable, with a few occasional rises. He had lost fifteen more pounds from the second surgery. I would come to realize that as the pounds were lost, his optimism would plummet; it was almost in direct ratio.

About a week later, we had a terrible day. I thought things had been going too well and found myself waiting for the crunch. I had tried not to anticipate the negative, but the apprehension and watchfulness were constantly with me. Early in the morning I heard Ray calling me urgently from the bathroom.

He had awakened soaking wet and thought that one of the bags had leaked. But this wasn't the case. The small incision where the abdominal catheter had been located following the first surgery had been left open after the second surgery for minor drainage. It was suddenly apparent why he had been running the fever when I saw the signs of infection gushing from the site. Every time he moved, it drained profusely, and it had startled and frightened him.

Miraculously, I was able to react calmly. I started to help him clean up, remarking, "Better an empty house than a bad tenant," and we both started to laugh. It certainly was better that the infection wasn't housing itself inside and remaining like a bad tenant. The little joke eased the situation some, and I called the surgeon.

I took Ray to the doctor's office during lunchtime, between appointments. He walked in with a big turkish towel stuffed in his pants. It was good that he still had his sense of humor. The doctor felt it was better that the infection was draining than to close the incision, so he put a tube back in to control the draining. Ray's fever broke shortly afterward and stayed normal over a week. However, the tube needed irrigation, and it would be a constant source of problems from that time forward. The three weekly irrigations and cleanup were the only things Ray ever objected to vehemently throughout his illness.

Throughout March, Betsy and Cindy usually stopped over in the evening after work, and Holly was a constant visitor. Some nights everyone came for dinner. Ray enjoyed the grandkids when he was up to the hubbub. During that week Gina called from Mexico to check on her father. We all thought of spring being just around the corner, but there was still snow melting on the ground.

A week later Ray checked in at the surgeon's office. Things looked fine except that his red count was down again and that meant more transfusions. We didn't get upset about that any more because he usually felt so much better afterward.

It was around this time that I became extraordinarily sensitive about minor things. This was foreign to my basic nature. But that day at the office the secretary and the nurse at the front desk told me that I couldn't go into the examination room with Ray. I questioned them, and they answered coldly that this was their policy. I could not understand their reasoning; I had been in the back only a week ago when we had come in with the towel hanging out of Ray's pants. I had helped the doctor with the irrigation in the back room and had done better with the situation than a young nurse who had become upset. Being able to assist Ray and the doctor helped me to feel useful, but the nurse remained adamant in her position. Tears choked me, and I was distressed because they had taken Ray away from me again, closing me out. This time it seemed totally unfair and unnecessary.

Later, I realized that this situation of being shut out, having no control, had duplicated in miniature what my life had become. The situation had affected me so deeply because it encapsulated all of the anxiety, pain, and helplessness of the past two months. It wasn't too hard to figure out, I thought, as I went over the feelings I'd experienced in the office. I spoke to Ray about it, and he was angry, too. He hadn't realized what had happened. "I'll speak to the doctor," he told me.

Next morning I dropped Ray off for a transfusion. He told me to come back for him. The thought of entering the hospital now made me so anxious that I became nauseous. At the start of his illness, I was always terribly uneasy going into the hospital. I guess I associated it with the beginning of the cancer diagnosis. Then, when Ray was so awfully ill during the second surgery, the hospital represented security to me. Now that he had been home awhile, my feelings shifted back to not wanting to go near the hospital again. Ray realized but perhaps didn't fully understand my dilemma. He let me off the hook, though, saying, "It's no big deal. I sleep through it anyhow." I felt guilty about it, but I just couldn't handle my anxiety.

When I came back to pick him up, he told me I had missed Dr. Thomas. He had been there over an hour talking with Ray. I was sorry that I had missed him. Then I thought that perhaps it was meant to be that way, just between him and Ray. I still believe with conviction that there are no coincidences.

Dr. Thomas had given him excellent news and a cause for celebration. He was ecstatic that the chemotherapy drugs were working, as well as amazed and excited that they had worked so rapidly. He called Ray a "textbook" case, meaning that specific results did follow specific treatments. He initially thought it would take at least six chemos to see any real progress, but Ray had shown positive results after just three. The chemotherapy treatments had cleared out the gel-like fluid that spread the cancer cells.

Ray was excited that the drug had stopped the cancer from spreading into two of the locations that he had seen in his island meditation. Dr. Thomas had been able to steer some-what into Rosemary's Alley, but that devastated area, the site of the original cancer growth, needed another barrage. Ray realized how accurate his meditation had been and was ex-cited about it, but still wouldn't mention it to the doctor. He told me later that he felt its purpose was for confirmation and reassurance that the doctor was on the right track.

He told me that he and Dr. Thomas had a long, serious conversation about his illness and what he had been through. I waited to see if he had anything more to tell me, but he was silent. He would share with me what he wanted. I was de-lighted that Ray was on such a high from it. He had developed a close rapport with Dr. Thomas and was fond of him. I was surprised that Dr. Thomas had allowed himself to get this intimate with Ray, but thinking back to the reading with Josef and what he had said about their past relationship, I under-stood why.

I wondered how the doctor was able to tolerate seeing such appalling sickness every day. One evening during Ray's first surgery, I had come into the hospital to speak to him and found him sitting in the lobby sorting papers while he waited for me. He looked tired and worn out. I could almost see the weights on his sagging shoulders. I asked him how he dealt with this kind of trauma day after day.

"Yes," he confided, "it's very, very difficult, but sometimes I do get an occasional miracle and that makes it all worth-while."

During Ray's second surgery in early March, I met a lovely nun in the hospital chapel. I had been raised Catholic and still occasionally returned to the church as an adjunct to my meta-physical pursuits. Edgar Cayce himself often advised people to return to the churches of their youth. That January, however, a visit to my local parish priest just didn't yield the kind of support I needed. When I met Sister Maria, she helped me regain a much-needed new perspective on those in religious life.

Because of my spiritual studies, my beliefs were quite different now from what I had been taught as a child. Even as I learned about alternative philosophies, I never felt that they conflicted with the teachings of the church; rather, I thought that they enhanced the basic teachings. I firmly believed in the concept of reincarnation—that after death, your soul returns to earth to inhabit a new body. The principle was recounted over and over to my ears during the sermons and the reading of the gospels. I discovered similar lessons often in the scripture. I saw the Law of Cause and Effect in Galations 6:7, where Paul wrote, " . . . whatsoever a man soweth, that shall he also reap." A previous life also seemed implicit in John 9:2, when Jesus was asked about a man who had been blind from birth, "Master, who did sin, this man, or his parents . . . ?"

My faith had always been in a loving God. I couldn't believe that He expects us to achieve perfection in one lifetime. Cayce's work had helped me see reincarnation as the key to understanding the apparent inequalities at birth. It also helped me understand the Bible in a new, deeper, helpful light.

I didn't say all this to Sister Maria, but we did have a stimulating conversation about religion. As we spoke together one morning, she kindly confirmed for me that I still had strong faith and believed deeply in God. With a smile she said that this was all I really needed. I saw her often at the hospital. I was grateful for her calmness and her interest in Ray's progress.

Toward the end of March the hospital called and advised us there was a problem with our health insurance. This was all we needed. When Ray was laid off from the large corporation, he had extended his personal health insurance, planning on using that until he found a new job. This extended insurance was not as comprehensive as what we formerly had, but we felt it would be sufficient for an interim coverage. I didn't know what the problem could be, but I knew we couldn't pay the astronomical bills that were coming in from the hospital at such an alarming rate.

Ray had traveled to work for years in New Jersey across the river, and the corporation had been pushing him to move there. He had resisted, however, because we were set up in Pennsylvania, with the kids in school and both our mothers living in the area. In January of 1985 the corporation came down hard and told Ray that we had to move. We sold our home in February of 1985 with plans for a May closing. Ray was laid off two months later, and the buyers would not forego the sale. We had rented a house with plans to live in it for a year until Ray found another job. He started his new job with the Boston company on January 1 of 1986. Two weeks later he underwent his first surgery.

I realized immediately that the new insurance had only been in effect for two weeks and wouldn't cover him, so we fell back on the extended insurance. I was concerned constantly about finances. We had to dig into the money from the house sale because of his layoff. We had tried to keep any other savings intact. The bills upset Ray terribly. When I finally got through to the insurance people, all they could tell me was that we had a unique situation and that they would try to accommodate us. It seemed that there was a question as to when the cancer actually began.

Palm Sunday came early. The weather was lovely and clear, but bitter cold. I hadn't attended mass in a while, and the procession with palms, commemorating the last days of Jesus, made me think about Him and what He had knowingly faced on that Palm Sunday so long ago. It was inspiring and suddenly impressive to me to realize that thousands of years later this celebration continues. Jesus' influence on the world is felt as strongly today as on that first Palm Sunday.

Gina and Brian returned home from Mexico in the afternoon, and Brian would be going home to Northern Ireland a day later. We were happy they were back, and it made the Palm Sunday weekend brighter.

Ray's appetite picked up, and he was feeling better. The doctor said they were hoping the tumor in the Alley (as we called it) would seal itself off and that the bacteria leaking in, causing the infection, would stop. The irrigation was taxing on Ray; he hated it, but it was necessary.

Easter was just around the corner, and I welcomed spring. We drifted along that week, from day to day, and I thought about our choices—our personal choices as well as the spiritual ones we make before we are born. As I endured my daily emotional confusion throughout that period in our lives, I never lost sight of my core beliefs that each soul incarnates, choosing freely its own spiritual mission with the highest intentions of fulfilling that particular mission on its journey back to God. Sometimes souls move forward immensely; sometimes they get stuck for numerous reasons and must come back lifetime after lifetime for balancing. I believed that one can go many lifetimes not fulfilling contracts made previously with God, with others, or with their own souls. Free will determines how we move and when we move. Then there may come a lifetime of monumental achievement for the soul when its mission moves to completion and it triumphs spiritually.

I knew that I had contracted with Ray before, probably in many lifetimes. I believe that we are in control of our destinies, but still I wondered how I might avoid drinking the cup that was being handed to me. I kept asking the Holy Spirit to send me a dream that would give me some insight into what my life had become, to help me close the gap between my spiritual truth and what my emotions were telling me.

It was Good Friday. I thought of Jesus again, His trial and death. I thought about how highly evolved a soul Jesus was to have taken on such a mission. I also thought about those who had been involved in the crucifixion. I could relate to Mary and her sorrow.

Easter turned out to be a beautiful day. My faith was replenished at church that morning, and I started out once again with a new burst of hope that God would cure all.

Chapter Six

Progress

(April)

On the last day of March Dr. Thomas had good news and bad news. The chemotherapy had stopped the spread of the cancer, but it hadn't stopped the cancer output from the original growth. Ray would have to have another chemo treatment immediately. They had been delaying this treatment since his bout with the infection, but now the surgeon advised Ray that he was caught in a vicious cycle. A direct channel had opened from the colon to the drain site and into the abdomen, resulting in a contained infection.

The perforation in the colon was about the size of a dime. Each new antibiotic was wiping out the germs leaking in through the colon, while another more resistent bacteria was replacing it. Ray's white count was down, indicating that the infection was contained, and the red count was up, showing that the red blood cells were working as they should. However, his resistance was low. The chemo would lower it further, leaving him open for yet another infection.

To make matters more complicated, his lungs were still susceptible to anything that came along, germwise. He was on a merry-go-round that just wouldn't stop. There was a risk either way: to let the infection continue or to go with the chemo, trying to shrink the tumor in the colon so the perforation would close itself. What had saved him so far was his body's natural walling off of the infection. I was amazed how the body compensated and protected itself, but Dr. Thomas wanted Ray back on the chemotherapy immediately. With that advice, Ray decided he had no choice but to go back onto the drug. We now realized that Ray's only hope was that the chemo would shrink the tumor at the cancer site.

That Tuesday night I decided to attend Annmarie's study group for the first time in months. I hadn't been able to handle much more than just getting through the day so that I could keep Ray company at night. I hadn't been able to meditate properly or with any regularity since January. My focus and concentration were nil. No matter how I tried to pull my mind into the light, it just didn't work.

Back in January I had tried to push myself into meditation, but it frustrated me so much that I had laid it aside. I prayed and talked to God every night and sporadically during the day, too, but only rarely could I sit for any length of time to meditate. Still, I felt deeply connected to spirit through that time and, looking back, I knew that spirit was my constant support.

I thought I would give meditation a try again that night. Maybe the change of pace of being out of the house would help me. Gina stayed with Ray while I was gone.

At Annmarie's, we prayed for Ray. The group held hands and joined together in a healing prayer circle. Annmarie led us as each person visualized white light and passed it clockwise around the circle. We could all feel the energy increase. Then we visualized Ray in the middle of the circle and held him in the healing light. Annmarie asked that Ray receive the light for his highest soul purpose. I visualized him clearly in my mind's eye and bathed him in white light from head to toe.

That particular evening we generated so much energy around the circle that each of us clearly felt it. It had physically manifested as a "revved up" feeling. All felt a tingling in our skins; our hands were soaking wet. Everyone in the group had been able to visualize Ray clearly and felt that he had taken the light we offered him.

During a break, I spoke to a member of the group, Bob, who practiced a healing technique called Reiki. He had just completed his training and promised to work with Ray. I reminded myself to get more information about Reiki and to see if there were any classes being offered in the area.

Ray was still meditating every morning, his own way, and it helped him relax, fight his depression, and free himself of the need for mild drugs for controlling his aches, nausea, and discomfort. I had bought him some meditation tapes with soft music, ocean and wind sounds. They helped him stay focused. He told me how much his meditation continued to help him concentrate on his inner self. He was now able to control his visualizations and to consciously picture his trips to his inner island. Whatever he was doing, I saw results and knew that this was right for him.

Ray's appetite was better, and the irrigation seemed to be helping with the drain site, which continued to be his biggest problem. He was anxious to get back onto the chemo to see if the drug would shrink the tumor and close the perforation.

A few days later, Bob and his friend Sally stopped by the house to administer a Reiki treatment. Before they began, I asked them to tell us a little bit about Reiki. I knew that it was being used in alternative healing techniques and that it was becoming widely known for the positive results it brought. They told me that it was a healing technique that originated in Japan. In Reiki, the basic concept is that there is a subtle system of life-sustaining universal energy circulating through and around all living physical bodies. This energy is called "ki" (pronounced *key*). The condition of your ki depends upon the harmony or disharmony experienced daily by your body-mind. If someone is sick, that person's ki needs restoration from the unpolluted source, which is God. You can be trained in Reiki to contact that unpolluted source and direct it to specific body parts. In many alternative healing techniques such as Reiki, the healer is only a passive instrument who conducts the energy. Ray and I listened carefully and found the entire concept fascinating.

Bob proceeded to lay his hands on Ray, making direct physical contact on different places of his body for about five minutes each. Ray immediately felt heat where Bob placed his hands. Bob did this in the area of Ray's lungs, drain site, and left side where the large tumor resided. Ray was amazed at the amount of heat created. He also observed how much more intense the heat was in the area of the large tumor.

There was a distinct and noticeable change in Ray's mood from this session, and he told me how good he felt. He said the relief from discomfort was almost immediate. The added reward was the lifting of his spirits, bringing him both inner and outer peace. I noted at the time that the effect lasted for about six hours. I was immediately aware that this time was longer than the effects of his meditations. Reiki seemed to give him fast, powerful relief almost immediately. I made up my mind to experience a Reiki session myself.

Incredibly, Ray slept straight through that night and was up early the next morning. He had no fever for the first time in weeks, feeling well enough to get out of bed and go down to the 7-11 for his paper and coffee. The visiting nurse came early and did the irrigation, noticing that the drainage was less than usual. Ray told me he felt a great change since the Reiki session last night. I asked him what he meant by a "great change," and he said, "I'm lighter. Not down. I just feel better all over." We decided to continue with his visualizations and meditations, but also to add Reiki. I would try to find out where Reiki classes were being given, so I, too, could learn how to use it.

Bob called later that day to offer Ray another treatment

before his next chemotherapy. I told him that I was waiting for Dr. Thomas to call with the scheduled date. He called almost immediately after I hung up. Dr. Thomas said that the surgeon confirmed that the tumors had shrunk somewhat from what he had seen during the first surgery. They were both pleased with Ray's slow but steady progress.

The following morning Ray was up and about early. He felt good again and discovered that his temperature was still normal. I allowed a quickening of hope to continue—not much, just a little. I dared not let myself get carried away. I wanted so much to let loose and pronounce that the healing had begun, but I knew I had better not. This was the worst part—allowing a trickle of hope to seep over the dam. It continued to be a cause of great anxiety, living in the gray area all the time. I wondered how Ray felt to receive something positive one minute, only to be knocked down again the next. He had always had good health and the faith that his body could heal itself. I thought then how we all take that gift for granted.

Ray felt better for nearly a week following the Reiki treatment, with no fever at all. Then one day toward lunchtime I saw the weariness suddenly return. It accelerated into overall misery and depression, which continued for the rest of the day—and the fever was back. Later in the evening he was able to meditate, which helped him feel a little better. My mind turned toward thoughts that perhaps I wasn't praying or believing enough. I, too, began to sink and decided if I prayed harder and had more faith, maybe I could change the course his body was traveling.

The chemo was scheduled for the middle of the week. I was concerned because of the rapid change in his temperament that day, but Ray was in no mood to discuss it. It was his decision to have the chemo scheduled. Yet the thought crossed my mind that if he didn't feel better in another day or two, I would tell the doctor my fears before allowing him to go in for the treatment. Even so, Ray knew the effects of the treatment much better than I did. All I knew was that I was weary of the rapid roller-coaster slides, falling like a rock off the top and plummeting to that depressing baseline.

Cindy had a reading with Josef around that time. He advised her that Ray was still making inner spiritual choices in regard to his physical condition. That meant his higher self hadn't decided whether to stay here or leave. I knew this to be true, but how hard it was. I told myself that tomorrow would have to be a better day.

April blew in her showers with full force. The weather the following day was cold, rainy, and miserable, contributing to the overall gloom we were all feeling. Ray had quite a bit of pain accompanied again by fever and was in a foul mood. I was looking forward to our Reiki healing session that night and hoped he would benefit as much as he had from the first one.

The Reiki session lasted about an hour. I took Ray's temperature afterwards and—wonder of wonders—it was normal. That was at about 8:00 p.m. We chatted awhile, and when Bob left, Ray was very peaceful, free of pain, and slept until 12:30 a.m. That's when I discovered that the discomfort had returned as well as a low-grade temperature. Despite this, I had definitely again seen immediate results that night from the Reiki in reducing Ray's pain and allowing him to sleep. I thought that even if Reiki were nothing more than mind over matter, isn't all healing in one way or another mind over matter? Weren't Jesus' healing miracles also mind over matter? The chemotherapy was scheduled for tomorrow, and I prayed that night that all would go well.

Morning found Ray feverish and miserable. We ventured out into the rainy, cold day to the surgeon's office for an examination. The doctor told him that the chemotherapy would be at 12:30 p.m. the next day. I checked him into the hospital later that evening for an overnight stay, and we hoped for the best.

Happily, the treatment went extremely well. When it was finished, Ray called me to come get him. He amazed me and everyone who heard him when he said, "Hurry up. I want to stop for a hamburger." The nurses laughed, astonished at his eagerness. It showed the astounding highs and lows, both physically and mentally, to which he was subjected. His spirits were up and his fever was down. This was a good combination. I had good news for both my friends, Joanne and Annmarie, who had been sources of comfort and solid support since January.

Even though it was April, the temperature was still in the 30s. Snow flurries had turned to hail and sleet, driven by a raging wind. Ray's fever was remaining down, but he was sweating a lot at night. He started to meditate again, surrounding the tumor with a silver blue light, and the pain dissipated. I asked him why silver blue instead of white light and he said, "Because I like blue, and the silver came in by itself." He told me that when he tried those colors this time, it made him feel lighter. The desolation lifted, and the discomfort went with it.

Three days after the chemo Ray felt good enough to go with me to pick up an old friend who was coming to visit. I always encouraged him to get out of the house if he was up to it. We had a nice, uneventful drive down, but coming back he got so thirsty we stopped for a cold drink. Evidently he drank it too fast, it made him nauseous, and we had to stop alongside the road until the nausea passed. I knew how upset he was, but he refused to complain. I wished that he would express more anger instead of keeping it bottled up inside. The ride had been too much for him, but because he was so headstrong, I didn't dare suggest it.

He couldn't wait to get home to meditate. His procedure now was when he felt rotten, he stopped whatever he was doing, did his meditation, picturing the silver blue light around the tumor, and he was able to stop any pain or discomfort. Sometimes I felt that he had a much better grasp of the situation than I did; sometimes I sensed that unconsciously he did know what was truly occurring.

The middle of April brought my birthday on Saturday the 13th, our granddaughter Sarah's First Communion on Sunday the 14th, and Gina's birthday and our 33rd wedding anniversary on the 15th. We decided to tie these events together. Ray sent me a beautiful bouquet of spring flowers on the 13th. Their aroma filled the entire room with sweetness. We planned to attend Sarah's First Communion followed by a party at Betsy's. Then we would celebrate the rest of the events during the week.

Early Sunday morning I looked out the window to see rain and cold and fog. I began to wonder if the real spring would ever arrive. But we wouldn't let it ruin our day, and it didn't. Before we left for the church to celebrate, Ray decided he couldn't handle both the church service and the party afterward. He opted to wait at Betsy's apartment, and Luke, who was three years old, kept him company.

The ceremony was lovely. The children all looked so shiny and wide-eyed with innocence. It was over too soon; everyone met in the back of the church and headed out. However, in the chaos, Betsy thought I was driving back with Cindy and Cindy thought I was driving back with Betsy, so I was left waiting at the church. I knew they'd realize as soon as they got to the apartment what had happened and come back for me. I was upset at first that I had been forgotten, but then we all had a good laugh about it. Ray felt good from the rest and enjoyed himself and the company at the party. When we arrived home that night, he had even more to eat. It had turned into a very good day, despite the weather. Maybe spring would bring healing and rejuvenation for him when she got here.

On the 15th, we celebrated Gina's 21st birthday and our

33rd wedding anniversary. It seemed the years had rolled by so quickly. It was hard to realize that our baby was 21, even more difficult to realize that Ray and I had been together almost a lifetime. I thought of the love and support the girls had given me throughout these last traumatic months and wondered how I would have managed without them. The years of love that Ray had given me were tucked deep into my heart. In the midst of our celebration, I thought that whatever happened that love was mine to keep.

The next morning we went out into gale-force winds and heavy pouring rain to keep an appointment with Dr. Thomas. Ray looked forward to seeing him and said he always felt better after talking with him. Dr. Thomas advised Ray that his condition was stable. After the blood report came back, he would decide about the next chemo. He prescribed different antibiotics to help the ongoing draining infection. When he got back home, Ray felt more emotionally elevated from the good report and was able to eat a decent lunch.

I loved big crystals and decided to hang one in the bedroom window. On those rare occasions when the rain stopped, the crystal grabbed the sunlight and reflected dancing rays of color onto the ceiling and walls of the room. The first time Ray saw it, he was surprised to see the silver blue color bouncing and spinning from the crystal. He remarked that it was the same color he had been using in his meditations to relieve pain. He was quite pleased and said he would try to focus on the crystal instead of his spot on the ceiling. He would funnel his concentration intently on the silver blue light from the crystal and transfer that light inside, directly onto the tumors. It greatly helped his focus, but he needed the sun to cooperate by sending its light through the crystal. Those meditations helped him tremendously in dispelling discomfort as well as in breaking the fever, which I'd seen occur time and again.

The next morning he told me that during meditation he

saw part of the lower colon, which had other perforations in it. Secretions were oozing from these perforations as well as from the tumor site. But the holding sack, as he had seen it, right by the tumor had less fluid in it. He said he saw silver blue light on the tumor, then he flooded the whole area with bright white light. He was going to try to zap it with the light now when he wasn't meditating, whenever he could get a quick image of the tumor. He went on to tell me that when he was finished with his meditation that morning, he was *free from all pain* and felt positive. He said he had gotten a great deal of relief before, but he continued to emphasize, "I mean no pain—not even a little discomfort. It was great!" I was ecstatic, because between the crystal meditations and the Reiki, I thought we might be able to keep his pain and resultant depression under control.

The following day was good for him. He was able to eat three times. His fever was consistently down and remained stable. Dr. Thomas called and scheduled the chemo for early in the coming week. However, Ray woke up the next morning experiencing severe pain and rigidity. Here we go again, I thought. I immediately called the surgeon's office. He told me to bring Ray to the hospital. Someone would meet us there.

One of the team surgeons examined Ray. When he was finished, he announced that he still felt Ray's condition was "status quo." The surgeon wanted to do some irrigation of the drain site, but Ray absolutely refused to allow it. He always felt so miserable afterward and had hated the procedure from the beginning. He decided to force the issue about discontinuing that activity. One of the other surgeons was examining him, yet Ray was so adamant about not doing the irrigation that the doctor let it go that day, told him to discuss the situation with the head surgeon, then we left. Ray napped after we got home. I called our friends to ask them to conduct a Reiki session.

How could we hit such highs and lows? We were riding the

roller coaster again, and the day had been very upsetting. The irony of it all was that today was finally clear, bright, and sunny, in the low 70s. My friends arrived later to administer a Reiki treatment. After they were finished, Ray felt relief. I contacted the Reiki group and asked when a few of us would be able to receive instructions. I knew it helped Ray, and I wanted to be trained so that I could do a session whenever it was necessary.

A few days later I awoke ill, with chills, aches, and fever. I wasn't ready to cope with this because Ray was due for his chemo that day, and I didn't want to give him anything else with which to contend. His immunity was so low that it was dangerous for him to be exposed to any sickness. I decided to stay in bed, behind closed doors, while Gina took him to the hospital and settled him in. He had a nice surprise from the admission office when he checked in. The insurance company had contacted the hospital; they would be paying most of the bills. He was thrilled and relieved when he heard that bit of good news.

The chemo went very well. I felt better that he was in the hospital that day and away from me until I could get the bug out of my system. He stayed overnight and came home the next morning.

We had recently read an article by Dr. Bernie Siegel of Yale University. His work proposed an emotional/mental link to the causes of cancer and also to its cure. That was the first time I had ever heard it stated so strongly. There had been hints at an emotional tie among other medical doctors, but Dr. Siegel's new book, *Love, Medicine, and Miracles* (Harper & Row, 1988), spelled it all out. I intended to order a copy, because I definitely agreed with him.

April was drawing to a close. We'd recently had some pretty good days. Ray was up and able to drive around a little more. He took short car trips to the bank and grocery store and other nearby places. His meditations kept him positive and free from pain. He was now using white, blue, and green lights in his visualizations, which helped him emotionally and soothed him physically. He had seen the green light emerge by itself during his meditations.

We had begun to learn more about various alternative healing techniques, when I met a healer named Shoshana. She was a third-degree practitioner of The Radiance Technique® (TRT), which, like Reiki, draws upon the power of universal spirit for energy. I made an appointment right away for her to visit Ray. She arrived promptly with her friend Michael to administer a treatment. Ray benefited greatly from the session, but felt it had been somewhat different with her. While she was treating him, he had drifting movements, seeing himself as a teen-ager, making decisions and plans, traveling here and there. He also saw himself and me in a small plane traveling over Ohio; it was extremely peaceful in the vast quiet sky. He felt he had drifted away into great calm and euphoria.

When he returned from this disconnected state, he was absolutely free of any discomfort and enjoyed the treatment thoroughly. Shoshana remarked that she was surprised that Ray gave forth such a vital life force and energy. It was extremely strong and quite unusual. She said that most of her cancer patients didn't project such a vital force.

After she finished working with Ray, she suggested that Cindy, her friend Cathy, and I be attuned to the universal healing energies. We weren't sure exactly what that meant, but we were willing to use whatever energy we could get! We felt that whatever the TRT brought to us could only be beneficial.

However, I wasn't prepared for what I received. Shoshana placed her hands about an inch above my head. I sat quietly and tried to clear my mind to attune to the universal energies. Suddenly I sensed a feeling of lifting. I had my eyes closed, but felt as if I were floating slightly above the chair. My hands had come together unconsciously in a prayer position. When I opened my eyes, my hands started to drift slowly upward. I thought I was going to lift up off my chair and follow them. Then, I consciously pulled my hands down, held onto the chair seat, and shut my eyes. Great multicolored spirals of light danced and spun and flashed behind my closed eyes.

Then Shoshana blew gently on my face. I thought of the age-old powers of the eternal, soft wind of spirit moving from the beginning of time. It felt like the Holy Spirit was being blown into my nostrils. I sensed that this experience triggered some ancient memory in me. I was completely calm when she finished.

Cindy wanted to experience anything she could. Because she was so sensitive, she was a little hesitant about completely opening herself in order to receive what she perceived to be an unknown. Michael placed his hands over her head. She felt like liquid was being poured right down through her. Cathy experienced deep warmth and peace. After Shoshana left, Cindy and I discussed what had happened to each of us and how we all felt so tranquil. We knew then how Ray felt after this treatment and agreed to schedule lessons in mid-May. Annmarie had expressed an interest also and contacted two teachers in New York who would come and instruct the four of us.

A few days later, the weather was bright, sunny, and much milder. I was praying that it would stay that way because Ray enjoyed sitting out in the back yard or on the front porch. He was able to take a few short business trips and started doing some work from home. I decided it would be good for me to get out of the house, too, so I took a temporary office assignment in one of the large pharmaceutical plants for two weeks. It went well, and I was happy to be out again. It distracted me from Ray's illness for short spans of time.

Ray continued to feel better, was out and about more. His red-blood cell count was good; his meditations and visualizations continued. He was now experimenting with the color orange and said that he saw the tumors breaking up; but it was hard to know if he was seeing past or future. Still, I decided at that point to allow myself to hope for a miracle again. Even a week or two of positiveness from him would give me the energy I needed to dare to be optimistic once more.

Ray's visualizing ability was truly wonderful; I started calling them visualizations rather than meditations. He would use the relaxation techniques that he had perfected for himself, then go into his visualization. When he would ask for the best color for healing himself, sometimes the color would come to him automatically. When the colors didn't present themselves strongly "on their own," he would consciously choose a color and visualize it.

Ray and I discussed colors after the first time he used the white light. He then decided he wanted to read something about colors and healing, so I gave him *The Ancient Art of Color Therapy*, by Linda Clark (Pocket Books, 1975). He enjoyed the book, which touched on the techniques of color therapy, and came to his own conclusion that he should ask for the most healing color at the time. I thought this was wonderful and didn't see where there was any need for him to learn about the deeper associations colors might have in connection with healing. Ray was doing well on his own.

In the past few months I had missed my own meditations, but my mind still couldn't focus, no matter how hard I tried. I had learned to meditate using colors as focal points and from the Cayce readings had learned that colors are associated with the body's spiritual centers, which the Hindus call chakras. The seven points are located throughout the body: at the base of the spine, the spleen, the solar plexus, the heart, the throat, between the brows, and at the top of the head. When I meditate, I visualize each of these centers, clear them if they aren't clean and bright, and open them as wide as I can. If I can't open a center in my visualization, then I know there is something blocking the energy associated with that point.

When I perceive these centers as being clear, I find I'm able to have a beneficial, refreshing meditation because the higher spiritual energy is able to flow freely. When I finish, I always draw the white light from a point two inches above my head downward, encasing my entire body in light for protection against negative outside influences. At that time I was obviously experiencing some blockages that were difficult for me to clear.

It takes time and tenacity to achieve ease in meditating without it becoming a chore, yet Ray had created his own system—practically overnight. He had brought the colors in on his own and, without realizing it, used them to focus his mind. He visualized the bright colors easily; they were working for him. Much as I wanted to share my knowledge of the spiritual centers with him, once he had his own effective method, I knew it was tailored specifically for him. He just wanted to get into his abdominal area and go to work. I didn't want to deter him from his own purposes with a lot of additional information.

The next chemotherapy went extremely well. Ray called me from the hospital the following morning to pick him up. He sounded positive and said he had some good news. When I arrived, he was dressed and ready to go. He told me that he had had a long talk with Dr. Thomas, who told him that his CVA (cancer count) had really taken a nose dive after the last chemo. It had been on a slow downward curve, but this time it had dramatically plummeted.

This was great news. We hugged each other with excitement. Ray was smiling and laughing. It took me a minute to fully comprehend what this new blessing really meant. It was the first piece of tangible scientific evidence we had that he was improving. Ray said that he attributed this to his meditation's reenforcement of the chemo drug. He was firmly convinced that by surrounding his tumor with the same silver blue light reflected through the crystal, he had broken the tumor up into tiny pieces. "I thought you said you only zapped it," I remarked. "Zapped it, hell!" he answered. "I blew those suckers away!" and he laughed.

It was marvelous to know that his inner meditations were accurately reflecting his physical progress. I didn't know if he had truly broken them to bits, but he had done something to the tumors to drop the cancer count. That drop in the count also meant that he had stopped the high production of cancer cells at the original site.

After that Ray felt so up and so much better physically and emotionally that he was inclined to overdo. The following days he was in and out of the house a great deal and drove short distances. Then he really did himself in by putting a tricycle together for Luke. He had to rest for a few days, but he reminded me that what the doctor told him, he had already known. He knew that he had broken up the tumors, but he wasn't sure how that would be reflected in the tests. He had seen everything ahead of time. Still, Ray said nothing about his meditations to Dr. Thomas.

I had bought a new juicer, but it just sat on the counter unused. Ray was never big on vegetables, yet I thought perhaps this would be a good way to get some into him. But he had refused any kind of vegetable juice that I tried. A few days later—I guess I was too eager—he really yelled at me about pushing food on him. He said he felt like a guinea pig for everyone's experiments. I couldn't understand what had triggered that outburst. Then a little while later, it came out that he had misweighed himself and had really lost five pounds, not gained them. He was upset and had projected his anger onto me. After we talked about it and he told me how upset he was over the weight loss, he calmed down. We decided to try a routine of four smaller meals a day instead of three. However, he quickly found out that a routine eating habit wouldn't work because he could only eat when he was hungry, and that fluctuated from day to day. But I was glad that his overflow of anger had cut itself loose.

His anger about the weight loss and things in general continued a day or two longer. At the next visit, Dr. Thomas assured him that it was expected to be up and down with the weight. However, both Ray and he were pleased with his overall steady progress.

Ray's meditations continued but always in a positive way. He disconnected so easily that I sometimes thought he had access to some private refuge in another time and place. This became part of Ray's daily routine, then; he told me he would be lost without it. Around that time he saw reddish-brown stuff in the tumor area and felt that the large tumor was still breaking up.

Two of the grandchildren came down with a virus and the doctor felt that was what Ray had over a week before when his appetite was off and he was feeling so bad. Ray had acquiesced with the irrigation after speaking with the surgeon, but he still hated it. The nurse came as scheduled and did an irrigation. The fluid was brownish, as he had seen in his meditation. It didn't surprise him because he had been right all along about the inner images that had been revealed to him.

CHAPTER SEVEN
AWAKENINGS

(May)

At the beginning of May, I joined Cindy, Cathy, and Annmarie in our first Reiki lesson at Annmarie's house. The class engaged in detailed discussions on the history of this art and on how "ki" flows. We also received instructions in the basic tecnhiques, such as how to place our hands on the recipient's body. We learned, as all novices do, that we would only be passive instruments through which the ki passes.

Toward the end of the class our instructors, Julie and Kate, gave us what would be the first of three attunements. It would be a different kind of attunement than I had received from Shoshana, because she had only balanced my energy. These attunements, we were told, would open the pathway for us to the unpolluted energy source.

Being only beginners, we weren't given an explanation as to how the attunement is called in from the universe. I had had such a wonderful balancing by Shoshana, however, that I was anticipating another pleasant spiritual experience. The thought of being able to access such powerful energy for the purpose of helping others was inspiring to me. I sat back, tried to clear my mind through relaxation, and made myself ready to receive something extraordinary from the universe.

The four of us sat in a row of chairs and were attuned two at a time. The instructors held their hands an inch or two above our heads. I immediately felt a calmness spread slowly from my head down through my entire body. With my eyes closed, I saw a large golden cross, brightly lit, which remained for a long moment in my inner vision. Then I experienced complete tranquillity, feeling as though I had been washed clean inside.

It was a pleasant, peaceful attunement. I was truly amazed at the calm feeling it had given me. After the four of us received our first attunement, we ate a light lunch, then continued with our discussions until it was time for our second attunements. I decided to go into the second one as I had the first—relaxing completely, which had now become much easier. I hadn't been able to enjoy such a level of physical tranquillity in months. Then, the second attunement began. As the instructor started to work over my head, I concentrated on her alone, opening my mind to her presence and trying to think of nothing but receiving love from the universe. As the attunement continued, I was alert, at peace, and calm. I was able to prevent my mind from drifting into any side thoughts.

Suddenly I received a clear vision. I was standing on high rocky cliffs looking down onto a large barren plain. Slightly off to the right, in mid-air, I saw a gigantic, transparent tornado. As I stood fascinated, watching this vortex of energy, I noticed that it was hourglass-shaped and wasn't carrying any debris. It swirled and whistled with a great sound; its tremendous energy was as powerful as any force of nature. I felt like a tiny bug from where I was standing and watching it. I couldn't understand why the tornado didn't touch down. It spun in one place, almost stationary, except for the movement of the hourglass itself. Then the scene shifted, and I was in the deep indigo of outer space, the darkness lit by thousands of stars and a quiet soft vacuum engulfing me. Huge tinker-toy-shaped objects, all hooked together, floated by me, reflecting their own light in the vast darkness as they tumbled and rolled and moved soundlessly overhead. As I stood and watched, they turned into giant blocks with letters and symbols written on them. Then, the whole scene faded, and I opened my eyes.

I was amazed at what I had seen; it made no sense to me. I was silent, overcome, and decided not to discuss it until I had a chance to think about it. That marked the end of that day's session. I decided to read more thoroughly *The Reiki Factor* (Radiance Association, 1985), by Barbara Ray, and the other material we had been given. Later, when I discussed the event with Annmarie and Cindy, they told me they had experienced some powerful feelings, too, which they couldn't quite explain. After this, we were wondering what would happen during the third and final attunement scheduled for the next day.

That night I read the book and other pamphlets because I hadn't had time to read them during class. I noticed some drawings and information in one small brochure. It was a picture of a spiral (double helix) of energy. I stared at the picture and suddenly realized that that was what had been presented to me in the form of a clear, almost transparent tornado, magnified 1,000 times. When I told Cindy about the tinker-toy-shaped objects turning into blocks with symbols on them, she suggested that it might have represented the DNA molecule and its component building blocks of the genetic code. My understanding seemed to fall together, then, and I knew that the purpose of my vision was to show me that ki is a natural part of the universe. I immediately sensed that it parallels the power of spirit that I had encountered in my cosmic dream.

After the first attunement, I had been left with a feeling of tranquillity, but suddenly being able to perceive such powerful forces was a little unsettling. When I was finished reading, I found myself wanting to meditate to quiet my mind. I needed to refocus; surprisingly, meditation now came easily. I began by opening the base chakra and, when I reached the throat, flashes of blue, like small bolts of lightning, dashed across the image of my throat chakra. From somewhere inside came the message, "You wanted the connection; you have your connection. So be it."

I knew exactly what that message meant. My beautiful transcendent dream of February flooded my mind once again with glorious images. How thankful I was that I had been able to bring back conscious memories of my cosmic home and that these memories had remained so vivid. The message was to remind me that I had already been given the connection; now I was being told that I should draw strength and energy from it.

During my attunement I had been shown powerful forces of nature and reminded that I was only a tiny part of my true essence, that the fragmented part of me was a member of the whole. I was almost euphoric while reliving my visit to the heart of the cosmos. But suddenly I felt resistance within me. Just as quickly, I seemed to become cautious about being in close touch with such unearthly phenomena. I told the apprehension to step aside because for Ray's sake I was determined to continue.

The changes that the attunements caused didn't stop there. When I opened my heart chakra, I was again impressed with unusual experiences. From somewhere deep in my inner memories, I was shown an image of myself being trained to do some sort of healing technique in ancient times. I felt literally pulled into a scene where I was one among a large group of men with shaven heads. We were dressed in white and listening intently to a tall, bearded instructor who was standing in front of the room delivering a lecture. We were sitting on wooden benches inside a small house with adobe-like white walls.

These new experiences were so exciting that it was difficult for me to go to sleep that night. I was by then eagerly looking forward to my third attunement. I had high expectations. But even though the insights I had received were positive, I remember asking that my next attunement experience be more gentle.

Annmarie's experience following the attunements had been somewhat different from mine. Where I had received visions, she had experienced more of a physical sensation. The instructor explained that psychically sensitive people have varying reactions to the attunements. Some receive insights and visions, as I had, and others experience physical effects. It was clear that what we had experienced had not been our imaginations. She explained the meaning of the double helix, a symbol of universal energy in the art of healing. She reassured us and told us that the last attunement would be successful as well.

Later in the morning, after more discussion and review, we started with the third attunement, two of us at a time, sitting in chairs as before. The instructor asked us to try to relax and put aside any distracting thoughts. We didn't have time to meditate, because, as before, she started immediately with the attunement. As I calmed myself physically, I called out to the Holy Spirit to help me settle down inside. I felt my whole body relaxing as I concentrated on the instructor's hands over my head.

Almost immediately, I saw a beautiful, large white water lily folded tightly onto itself, attached to its bright green pad. I felt that this was more like a vision because the image remained constant, independently of my will. I marveled at the stunning vividness of the exquisite colors I was seeing. The water lily was in the middle of a small tranquil pond. I saw the blue sky all around me, dipping down to meet the horizon. As I watched this peaceful setting, the water lily began to unfold, opening to the sun. Rising up out of its center were golden spirals of light and bright white flashing circles. I watched for a moment longer, then the vision faded. I felt so good and peaceful, so completely relaxed that I had to move or I would have drifted off to sleep.

This third attunement was beautiful. I had always associated anything white, peaceful, and serene with the Holy Spirit. I had asked the Holy Spirit for a softer scene, so I believe the Spirit had intervened for me. But even though the lily seemed serene, I had sensed great energy from the golden spirals of light and the white circles emanating from its center. It had reminded me that gentleness and peacefulness didn't mean softness in the sense of weakness. It was a serene and tranquil sight, Oriental in flavor, connecting nature and energy. I hoped it would help me to cope with my constant stress and eventually help Ray as well. I had seen the powerful force of the helix plus the gentler side of the lily. I thought I could use this beautiful scene by recapturing and focusing on it during meditation.

My vision of the water lily sparked my memory of another scene of something white and peaceful. Years before, I had attended a seminar on shamanism. In meditation we had been instructed to discover our power animal archetype—the animal that best symbolized our source of strength. Most of the people in the group had received powerful images of mountain lions, eagles, hawks, and even a porcupine, so I felt a little foolish when I announced that I had seen only a white dove. The instructor told me that it was a beautiful symbol, but everyone else just looked at me sideways, not knowing what to make of it.

Not until later did I realize the full significance of the white dove, a universal symbol of the Holy Spirit. Like the others at the seminar, I, too, had always associated power with physical strength. I had a difficult time reconciling within myself that spirit is also strength. In reading 262-29, Edgar Cayce said that "the Christ Consciousness is the Holy Spirit . . . " What, then, could be stronger than my dove?

After our third and last attunement, we were now first-degree practitioners. (To qualify as an instructor requires completion of three degrees.) We couldn't wait to practice on Ray. The first time Cindy, Cathy, and I worked on him, he almost fell asleep. He was amazed at the calmness it gave him, how it eliminated his emotional distress. I still wondered, though, why I continued to vacillate between the committed and the skeptical. There I was. I had actually seen Reiki work. I'd witnessed its beneficial emotional effects without a doubt. I'd seen it eliminate his fever and pain. I guess skepticism was my nature, even after all I had seen. Annmarie said it was good to be skeptical. It keeps us grounded and helps us hold on to our common sense.

A few days later Ray told me that he felt well enough to take a trip in the car to his office in Boston. I was hesitant, but he had decided that he definitely wanted to go. After we made the plans, we left, stopping to pick up Ray's associate who covered the New Jersey area. It was an extremely hot day for May, in the 90s, and we had to use the car's air conditioner. We stopped for lunch. Ray ate lightly, sleeping in the back seat the rest of the way.

When we reached the motel, however, he really felt lousy and had a slight fever. I administered a healing treatment, and miraculously his fever left. He was able to relax and had a sound sleep that night. He told me my hands on the painful areas of his body felt "hot" and alleviated the discomfort. He was much better the next morning, and things went well for him at the office. We were glad to arrive home after the long drive, but drizzle, terrible heat, and humidity welcomed us back into Pennsylvania.

It was chemotherapy time again, but Ray hadn't felt well during the last few days. Even after he checked into the hospital, Dr. Thomas wasn't able to determine the reason for this. He thought perhaps the tumors were growing again, but Ray's stomach was still soft. Then he suggested that maybe it was a holdover from Ray's recent virus. I was beginning to feel that too much was being blamed on a virus from several weeks ago.

Ray was weighed in, and we were all alarmed and disappointed when we saw that he had lost five more pounds. It was always upsetting to him when he had a weight drop because he tried so hard to eat. Dr. Thomas decided to keep him overnight and give him a transfusion, then go ahead with the chemo the next day. I began to have crazy negative thoughts. I wondered if the Reiki was helping him or, in fact, might be fast-forwarding the cancer to its conclusion. Of course, I realized later that this was impossible, but I suggested to Ray that maybe we should stop the treatments. He disagreed adamantly with me and said that they helped him too much, that he couldn't do without them. I was constantly grabbing at even the slimmest reason why his illness was progressing. True to my Aries nature, I expressed myself spontaneously and irrationally. I knew that the treatments were not contributing to his sickness, but my emotions were so sensitive that at times they knocked my logic for a loop.

Ray called that evening from the hospital, saying that he felt better after the transfusion and that he had eaten a complete dinner. The next day, the chemo went well. He announced that he was feeling 100 percent better. He also exclaimed that he was determined to put the weight back on.

By Memorial Day, I realized how the hours and weeks had blended together, having no dimension or solidness to them. Memorial Day brought beautiful mild weather, and our granddaughter Sarah had decorated her bike with red, white, and blue streamers to ride in the town parade. We watched it from our large front porch. Ray enjoyed all the kids and the local bands from his perch on the porch. The girls and Grandma Eva joined us in the afternoon for a cookout.

Gina finished her last semester on schedule and was contemplating a summer visit with her fiance in Ireland. She usually stayed with Brian and his family a few months in the summer because they saw each other infrequently during the year. But this time, she was torn between going to be with Brian and staying here to be with her father. I knew that she was having an extremely difficult time dealing with her father's illness for the last three months, but she also missed Brian terribly. Ray saw how hesitant she was about leaving, and he told her to go. "What can you accomplish here? I'll be all right," he said and truly meant that he wanted her to go.

I spoke with her alone and told her that if things suddenly got worse here I would call her and that Dad would feel better if she went. He really didn't want her sitting here all summer. Ray wanted to take her to the airport limo, which was at a local motel, a short ride from the house. We absolutely could not make the drive to JFK airport in New York.

Gina would be upset when she said good-by. I also knew how teary I would become when she left. Any kind of separation upset me at that time, but I figured I could muddle through. We dropped her off at the limo and quickly said good-by. I told myself that she would call and write and that she would be home again before too long, but I knew I would miss her.

Two days later Ray was miserable again. We had learned to expect this boomerang effect right after the chemo. The only answer was rest in bed until some of his strength returned.

It was around that time that Fluffy, my beautiful black-and-white long-haired cat, disappeared. We didn't let her out very often because she had become a house cat after being hit by a car when she was young. Her leg was broken in the accident and the resultant surgery involved a pin in her leg, keeping her in a playpen for six weeks, then more surgery to remove the pin. She had become an important member of the household and I loved her dearly.

She liked to come out in the back yard with us. The day before, when we had gone out, she cried to join us so I let her.

Then she just vanished. We searched all over but couldn't find her. I wouldn't let myself contemplate at that moment that she could possibly be lost. I told myself that she would show up. I wouldn't accept the fact that anything this cruel could happen to me then.

The next day Ray felt a little better. Then Dr. Thomas called and said that the lab had found an abnormality in one of his lungs. He didn't tell me what it was, only that it was an abnormality. He wasn't sure, but he thought this was what was responsible for Ray's recent fever and pain. The doctor prescribed Percoset for pain and told Ray to rest over the upcoming weekend. I refused to let my mind run wild with that awful word "abnormality," because I could easily focus on it and drive myself crazy. I decided to just let it lie there. I'd found that I was becoming quite adept at controlling my thoughts.

Two days later Fluffy finally turned up. She had gone under our old house and gotten caught. I was in the back yard calling her, as I had been doing for the past two days, when I suddenly heard a little meow. At first I couldn't figure out where it was coming from, but then I heard her again. I got down on my knees, pulled aside a block of stone, and there she was! I hugged her to me tightly; something had finally gone right. She was extremely hungry, but since she was quite fat, she was none the worse for her ordeal. I vowed never to let her out of the house again. Later that day Gina called from Ireland and told us it was 58 degrees there and rainy. We were sweltering in 92-degree heat. It was unusual to have such a cold April and such a heat wave one month later.

We found ourselves praying that Ray would gain some weight. He kept losing, five pounds at a clip, and he had become quite thin. We treated him daily and it still calmed him, taking away his discomfort to the point that he never needed the Percoset. However, his weight kept falling. He seemed to be going downhill in a slow, steady decline. We didn't know what else we could do for him. I sensed that something had happened in his inner self, but I had no idea what it was.

The next morning brought absolute disaster. Ray woke up with a high fever and chills. Dr. Thomas wanted him in the hospital immediately. We met the doctor in the emergency room and he had bad news. The cancer count had come back from Princeton labs; it had risen dramatically. Ray's stomach had become swollen and rigid on the right side again, and Dr. Thomas didn't like that either. He told us that evidently the chemo drug had stopped working, which sometimes happens. Ray had reached the drug's saturation level.

I was stunned for the moment at the deluge of terrible news. I thought I should be able to handle the downhill plummet after all the roller coaster rides we had taken. But each plummet down was just like the first. From previous experiences it didn't get easier but became increasingly more difficult. I still found I couldn't rapidly adjust my emotions to accommodate the ever-changing aspects of his illness. Less than six weeks before we were experiencing joy at the good news from the lab. We had been riding on that last news item of the fantastic drop in the cancer count. The present news, however, was horrendous and had devastated us.

Dr. Thomas continued, saying that he wanted to try a new drug. I can remember our exact conversation. He explained that it has more side effects. However, he said, because Ray had done so well on the previous drugs, he was anticipating that the side effects from the new drug would be minor.

"What do you mean by minor side effects?" I asked him.

"Nauseousness is the biggie," he said. "I've had good results from this new drug with people who have become immune to the first medication."

Then I finally pinned him down and asked, "What will we do if the drug doesn't work?"

He hesitated for a moment, then leveled his eyes with

mine. "There are some other alternatives," he softly said, "but if nothing works, Ray has two to three months at most."

It was finally out in the open like a raw wound, but at that moment I was only letting the information in at the top level, intellectually. I knew that I'd eventually be hearing this but hadn't allowed myself to ask those kinds of questions before. I decided then to go ahead and ask him all that had been rushing through my mind.

"How will this happen?" I asked.

"Infection, blocked bowels, renal failure, and other things," he said.

His words lay on the air between us. I wanted to push them back at him, not accepting what had come to me from him. He told me then that he was very sorry. I knew as I looked at him how genuinely upset and disappointed he was.

"Ray has amazed me with his recuperative powers," he said sadly. "I was hoping for a miracle and I have seen miracles. But I don't think I'll see one here."

Ray had heard none of this, and I asked Dr. Thomas how we would tell him. I sensed that Ray was already aware of what was going on, but it had to be said out loud.

"I'll speak to Ray about everything," he said, and the sound of sadness in his voice touched me deeply because it told me how truly sorry he was.

Dr. Thomas visited Ray a short time later and told him about the new drug, Platinol, and that he would like Ray to give it a try. He advised Ray to continue to be positive. There would be side effects, but he emphasized to Ray that because of his good handling of the first chemo drugs, he didn't expect severe effects. Dr. Thomas told me the drug was what they called a "heavy metal," and it was toxic. I was shocked by the words "heavy metal" and "toxic." I felt them to be horrendous and didn't want Ray to take it. But he was adamant and said he had no other choice. I felt he did have a choice; it was time to stop putting these foreign substances into his body. He would either be healed by his own processes with the help of God, or it was time to let nature take its course. But I kept that thought to myself at the moment.

It didn't make sense to me to put a highly toxic and poisonous drug into his already defenseless immune system. It could kill him. I didn't think there was any medical way to cure him at that point in time. If he was going to be healed, it would be on another level. He had given science every means, and it wasn't going to work. I didn't think the doctor had told Ray everything that he had said to me; also I didn't think it was right to discuss my fears with Ray. I had a lot of further thinking to do. My choice wouldn't be his, but then I wasn't walking in his shoes. He had to make his own decision.

Betsy, Cindy, and I met at the hospital to support Ray and each other after we heard this news that the present drugs were no longer working. After we left, Holly came by to see Ray. Later, Ray told me that she had lain next to him, sobbing, telling him how much she loved him and that she didn't want him to die. He said to her that he had no intention of dying.

My heart broke when I thought about the mental suffering Ray must have been going through in making this decision. I knew the doctor told him how serious things were and had given him the choice of the Platinol. Where did Ray get his strength and courage? His faith that he would be healed and his patience in waiting for that healing were something that I had never seen before. He was not denying that he was terribly sick, but he would not give up hope. He still believed in miracles. At that moment I wanted to feel some of his hope, that he would have a chance with the Platinol. Yet on the other hand, I could not ignore the truth I was receiving from within myself. I was caught between my inner awareness that he was probably not going to make it and trying to be supportive of Ray's faith and hope that he would eventually get well.

As we left the month of May behind us and moved ahead into June, it was still unbearably hot and muggy. Rachael,

Holly's older daughter, celebrated her third birthday on the last day of May. Ray was not well enough to join us on the hour's drive north to her house.

After we arrived, we went through the birthday party motions as best we could for Rachael's sake. We were all depressed and our thoughts were with Ray, but we continued on because the children didn't understand. It was Rachael's birthday and that was important. I had made her a teddy bear couple with all the matching clothes. I had done it for her and also to keep myself busy. She was delighted and played most of the afternoon with them.

I left before the party broke up, dropped Grandma Eva off, and hurried home to Ray. I was worried about him the entire time. When I arrived home, I found him touchy and depressed. He didn't want to talk to me at all; he was depleted and only wanted to sleep. Give me the strength to face the days ahead, I prayed. I was depressed and detached, though I couldn't even begin to imagine how he felt.

Ray had a profoundly calming dream that night and told me about it the next morning. He dreamed he was going to Crystal City, a lovely section of Washington, D.C. We were in the car together and driving through Virginia's Shenandoah Valley. He was going on a business trip to solve a technical problem for a customer. He told me in the dream that he used a "different" technique to solve it. He also felt very healthy in the dream. He knew he was physically sick and had the bags on his body, but, even though he was thin, he felt well.

He told me the scene shifted, and we were driving high up into the Berkshire Mountains in Massachusetts, because I had never been there before. We drove along a winding road and there was a river running through the countryside. A stream ran along the side of the road with tall evergreen trees marching beside it. He told me how beautiful it was.

I felt that, for him, this was a different kind of dream. In other recent dreams, he always found himself inside his body working with his illness. This traveling dream, however, seemed to offer a clear message. We discussed its interpretation together and agreed that our trip to Crystal City meant that it was definitely time for him to see his life as clearly as possible.

In order to reach that point, Ray had to drive through a valley (the earthly realm of his physical illness). The purpose of the trip was to solve the technical problem—the illness itself. He intended to use a "different" technique to solve it. I interpreted this as meaning a spiritual solution or some solution other than a medical one. He knew he was physically sick in the dream but felt well, meaning that he had experienced the dream from the perspective of his higher self.

After he decided to use this "different" technique to solve his problem, the scene shifted from the valley to the mountains, representing his access to the higher levels of consciousness. Ray drove along a winding road (the difficult path he was following in this life) and saw a river, the symbol of crossing to the other side or death. The river, however, was not in front of him but on the other side of the road. This told me, thankfully, that he was not yet ready to cross it. After we had finished discussing it, he agreed with the interpretation.

We were still giving Ray regular healing treatments, which continued to help him greatly. He announced again that he didn't think he was ready to "check out." I couldn't say a word because my throat was shut with the pain of grief. He told me he was not frightened of dying because he knew that there was something to look forward to afterward. I had always sensed that he believed this, but it was the first time he had ever expressed it. I hoped that by the act of verbalizing the thought, it would help him to move forward spiritually.

He was dreaming a lot lately but said he couldn't remember most of his dreams. I was suspicious that he was dreaming of information that he didn't want to share with me. Perhaps it was meant for him alone. Many of his dreams took place in a small blue and white airplane. As a pilot, Ray loved being up in the air experiencing freedom and weightlessness from the earth. No wonder he dreamed of flying. Flying, for him, had always meant freedom from the burdens he carried here. He seemed to be drawing some unexpressed benefit for himself through these dreams because he was constantly off somewhere in deep thought.

Not long after, he began to talk about all the unusual psychic experiences he'd had in the past few months. He was trying to put the events together, admitting that even though he wasn't able to grasp and dissect them logically, he was no longer able to deny them. He no longer cared whether his out-of-body experiences and what he was seeing in his meditations sounded "weird"—it was becoming his truth.

I sensed strongly that Ray's soul was making decisions on a deeper level, but at that point in time I wouldn't have been ready to accept that he had made a definite decision to leave me. Despite my dreams and the insights of my visions, my humanness constantly got in the way. Acknowledging that Ray might actually be leaving me brought me peace in one way, but in another I just could not bear the thought of it.

It was around that time that I picked up the book, *Death, the Final Stage of Growth* (Touchstone Books, 1986), by Elisabeth Kübler-Ross, a world-renowned psychiatrist known for her ground-breaking ideas on death and dying. Dr. Kübler-Ross, in "Omega," the final chapter of her book, tells us that our concern should be to live while we're alive, "to release our inner selves from the spiritual death that comes with living behind a facade designed to conform to external definitions of who and what we are." I thought how many of us live our lives conforming to others' expectations, thereby stifling our own spirits. Ray hadn't been able to break the bond from the childhood shackles of definitions that had conditioned him. Those shackles had suffocated his spirit, never allowing his inner core to break free into the light.

Despite how I was feeling that day, Kübler-Ross' words reenforced my belief that Ray was at last able to work from his own internal valuing system—an internal system that seemed to be connected to a great universal spirit, sending him knowledge in great quantities, enabling him to move into spiritual awareness for the first time in his life.

CHAPTER EIGHT
CHRISTINA APPEARS

(June 1-25)

The seven years that we lived in Florida had been both the best and the worst period in our lives together. The unhealed emotional baggage from my childhood had begun to cause havoc in my life. After Gina's birth, I became severely depressed and began to experience panic attacks. The shifting of hormones from the pregnancy had apparently triggered the attacks which were masking all the anger, guilt, and insecurity I had been suppressing for years. It was time for me to clean out my childhood house, so I sought help by way of therapy. Although "meeting myself" was the most difficult, painful task I had ever undertaken, this initiative eventually freed me from the past, enabling me to enjoy my life with a new perspective. Achieving freedom from my longtime conditioned reactions would allow me to rear my children with a more open perception than my parents had. It would allow me to break the generational chain of unenlightened upbringing.

Ray had been extremely supportive during that time and was always available when I needed him. He literally ran the house and took care of the children during my first year of therapy. But, when one partner in a marriage gains a new perspective, the partnership can become strained and unbalanced. As we discussed the changes I was going through, we knew that Ray, too, needed help with his own emotional blocks. So Ray decided to seek help as well.

I had been fortunate in finding a wonderfully perceptive psychiatrist, who I knew would be good for Ray, too. Ray began his sessions with him, but they only lasted a short time. Ray's childhood had been so traumatic that when he tried to relive it in therapy, it was more painful than he could bear.

Recalling that time twenty-five years before, I realized that at that juncture in our lives we had taken different paths. When Ray became sick, memories and symbols of Florida came up often in his dreams. This reenforced my belief that it had been a time when he made some critical choices for his life. Someone suggested to me that his choice not to heal the trauma of his childhood at that time is what planted the seeds of his illness.

He had simply been unable to bring those hidden childhood experiences out into the light to heal them. To his much-deserved credit, however, he later continued with his therapy in Pennsylvania, with a kind and loving psychiatrist who helped him achieve at least some breakthroughs in understanding himself. Still, he was never really able to dig down into that deep, painful, inner core of himself. He and I then tried to work on that core together. While I felt that he gained some awareness, he never had a complete understanding.

On the first of June we left for the hospital around 1:00 p.m. for Ray's first treatment with the new drug. Although the girls and I were anxious about it, Ray remained calm. He checked in, but when they weighed him, we were appalled to learn that his weight was down to 133 pounds. I was shocked to realize that he had lost a total of 60 pounds. In January, when this vile monster invaded him, he had weighed 193 pounds. He was 5'11"—no wonder he looked so gaunt and haggard. I swallowed back tears, seeing how his once strong body had been so ravaged.

He would have fluid pumped into his abdomen that night to dilute somewhat the Platinol they would infuse tomorrow. The cardiologist checked his heart and lungs, and the surgeon examined his abdomen. Dr. Thomas was being cautious because he knew how strong the chemo drug was. I didn't think my anxiety could escalate any further, but it continued to mount to an all-time high. I was beginning to realize that it wasn't the probability of his dying that was causing me such anxiety; it was the terrible way he was getting there.

Adding to this, I was focusing all my fears and anxieties onto the hospital itself. My displaced anxieties were causing me to associate the lifeless building with a devouring monster. All I knew was that I was terrified anytime I entered it. We got Ray settled in, and I left him in the hospital for the night, planning to come back in the morning.

I had a free minute, so I called the bookstore and ordered Dr. Bernie Siegel's book, *Love, Medicine, and Miracles*. I had known about the book for the last few weeks and read the great reviews it had received, but it was not out in the stores yet. I decided to call Dr. Siegel's Center for Exceptional Cancer Patients in New Haven, Connecticut, to find out what kind of work they were doing. The receptionist told me that Dr. Siegel would be lecturing in Allentown, Pennsylvania, only an hour away from where we lived, on June 20 and promised to send me some material, including a tape.

She told me about Dr. Siegel's therapy groups. I wondered if it would be possible for Ray to join one. It would be wonderful for him, but I felt that Connecticut would be too far for him to travel. I made a note on the calendar that night to tell the girls about the June 20th lecture date. I definitely planned to attend, and I was sure they would want to go, too. If it were possible, perhaps Ray could go, as well. It would be a "wait and see." I was looking forward to the book's arrival and the promised material from the Center.

I went to bed that night, dreading the next day, knowing what Ray would have to face, praying that all would go well.

Ray called early the next morning and told me that the treatment had already begun. "So far, so good," he had said. However, when Cindy and I arrived at the hospital, Ray started to experience terrible reactions to the drug. He was only semiconscious from the sedatives they'd given him but that didn't stop the traumatic physical side effects. He was vomiting severely and constantly and could not be left alone for a minute. The violent wretching went on and on. I felt absolutely helpless. There was no other medication that would help. Having to watch him being so sick was a devastating experience. Panic-level anxiety overtook me. I could no longer even pretend to remain calm. At 5:00 p.m. I had to leave the room because I knew I would soon lose all control and start screaming if I stayed a moment longer. Cindy was able to stay with him, so, blinded by tears, I groped my way out the door and over to the elevator.

I got down to the parking lot and just stood there shaking for a few minutes until my anxiety subsided. I leaned against the car and thought I had surely come up against my breaking point as I desperately tried to collect myself. That moment in time had been my dark night of the soul. I realized that nothing yet to come, not even death, could be as terrible as how I felt at that moment. Finally, I collapsed onto the front seat of my car, wondering if I could make it home. Why did he have to go through this torture? The day had turned into the worst nightmare of my life. Still immobilized, I just sat in the car. I could not believe that anything could be that awful; I thought Ray had already reached the height of unimaginable physical trauma. I wanted to run and run and never come back—but there was no place for me to go.

Somehow I managed to drive home. Cindy called later to tell me that after an hour or so, the severe reactions had begun to taper off. Ray was doing better now and, because of the sedation, hadn't remembered much, as the doctor had predicted. By this time I was ready to explode. My own nauseousness had taken over, and I didn't know what to do with myself.

I went outside and decided to walk with the dog. But somehow, my mind shut off every sight and sound that was trying to pry in. As I walked, I was only able to hear distant muffled noises. I had walked quite a distance before I realized my outer senses were starting to return. My ears were being raided by the sounds of summer around me. Birds were chirping night calls to each other in the soft descending twilight, the muffled buzz of a lawn mower droned far off, and excited shouting echoed from the baseball diamond in the small park.

The summer sounds invaded my senses then and were slowly converted into meaning in my head. The summertime smells of grass and flowers and the distinct odors that I associated with the warm times crept in. Colors penetrated my eyes and were translated into meaning. The bright greens of the lawns and the white houses with different-colored trims caught my attention. I came back. Where was all this going to end? If only I could have drifted off into summerland itself to float on and on . . .

There was only one reality, despite all of life unfolding around me that evening; I didn't want Ray to have to endure the effects of that drug again. It was disastrous.

I forced myself back to the hospital later that evening. Cindy had remained for most of the afternoon, then Betsy came to stay for awhile until I got there. They had all been so good, so strong. I felt like a deserter but decided not to dwell on that thought. I only stayed a short time because Ray wanted to sleep. Surprisingly he didn't look that bad. I thanked God that he was doing well because I wasn't able to stay at the hospital much longer that night.

The next morning I called Ray early. He told me that he was

doing better and to come over. He said the cardiologist would be in to draw off some fluid that had accumulated around his lungs to help him breathe easier. They wanted to check the fluid to see if it contained any cancer cells or if there was any infection.

When I arrived, however, Ray's room was empty. I panicked. I didn't know where they had taken him; his roommate thought down to x-ray. I raced downstairs to the x-ray area. The clerk told me that they were only taking pictures. I was relieved and went back to his room to wait. Shortly afterward, the technician wheeled him into the room. When the cardiologist arrived to draw off the fluid in Ray's lungs, my stomach turned over when I saw him prepare his equipment. I had to leave the room. But it only took him a minute to siphon off about a quart of fluid, and Ray felt immediate relief. He was then discharged, and we went home.

I sat beside the bed that night looking at Ray, and although it was nearly six months since he had been sick, my mind still couldn't accept what had happened. His once strong body had been depleted, and the traumas that he had suffered were devastating. Even though all that time had passed, for a fleeting moment I felt as if it were a nightmare and eventually I would wake up. Then, I told him that he was the bravest, most courageous person I had ever known, and he just smiled. I marveled at his fortitude and thanked God for giving him the stamina to endure such trauma. Ray's strength was unwavering and unending. Yet I thought again and again that I wished he would scream and curse and shake his fists. I knew I would never have had the emotional and physical courage that he continued to steadfastly reveal.

He slept most of the next day and was able to experience a successful meditation. During the meditation he saw some remaining fluid inside his chest. Because he got such a good feeling from using colors, he visually blasted it with white light. He truly believed that there was no fluid left after that and he told me plainly that it wouldn't bother him any more. Fortunately, his horrible chemo experience was not a vivid memory. He didn't realize at a conscious level how horrendous the treatment had been, and for that I was thankful.

Ray told me spontaneously that evening that he wanted to live to see his grandchildren grow up. He cried as he spoke, and I wept. He said that he wanted to tell his girls again how much he loved them all. He told me that he intended to make other changes in his life if he made it through. He'd be more open and communicative on all levels and would drop his work life to a lower priority. He'd try to understand and express where he stood in relationship to God in his life. Holly came in later, and we sat and continued our conversation. He wanted her there so he could tell her how much he loved her.

Finally Dr. Siegel's book, *Love, Medicine, and Miracles*, arrived. I rushed down to the bookstore to pick it up. I devoured the entire book that night. His advice to patients and caregivers alike was inspiring and direct, and I recommend it even now.

Dr. Siegel, a practicing surgeon at Yale University Hospital, helps people survive cancer. From working with many cancer patients, he observed that those who survive have certain characteristics in common. He calls them "exceptional patients." It seemed that these exceptional patients are able to take control of the healing process. They have the courage to participate with their doctors and actually influence the outcome of their illness. Dr. Siegel feels that it's necessary to examine the *role* illness plays in the patient's life and for patients to examine their attitudes about themselves.

The majority of Dr. Siegel's patients suffer from cancer, but his ideas can also be applied to other illnesses, such as multiple sclerosis, AIDS, arthritis, diabetes, and heart disease. The way to healing was the same. In 1978, Dr. Siegel founded the ECaP (Exceptional Cancer Patients) group, which involves the patient in both individual and group therapy to hasten personal change and healing. After he saw the dramatic results the patients achieved with his therapy, he wanted to spread the word to make others aware of their own healing possibilities. Like Edgar Cayce had said years before, Dr. Siegel acknowledged the connection between the mind and the body, breaking through many misconceived medical perceptions. He encouraged all of his patients to use that connection in healing themselves.

Included in the book were several excellent guided visualizations. Dr. Siegel suggests that patients make their own tapes, using the background music of their choice. He recommended soft, soothing music that did not distract from the visualization itself. The tape should start out with relaxation suggestions, similar to those one uses in meditation. It's remarkable that Ray was already using many of Dr. Siegel's techniques, such as visualizing his body and checking for illness from head to toe. But the new twist for Ray was visualizing himself as being physically well.

These suggestions are followed by a guided meditation in which the patient imagines himself or herself flying in air balloons, walking along a path, through gardens, along beaches, and across bridges, and finding chests with messages in them along the way. The patient imagines himself or herself walking through rooms in houses and then into the body to actively fortify the immune system. Finally, the guided meditation suggests that the patient meet his or her guide (some people felt it was their guardian angel or soul or higher self), and that the guide would help.

As soon as I read this, I ran to find my microphone and recorder. I couldn't wait to set up some tapes for Ray. There were a number of guided visualizations in the book, so the first tapes I made were exactly as written. In succeeding tapes, I varied places and activities but always followed the same themes as suggested, such as using Ray's individual health problems instead of the general health conditions depicted in the book.

Ray loved the tapes. Because he was already able to detach so quickly, he easily slipped into these visual journeys. (For those who feel unable to make their own tapes, pre-made tapes can be acquired by mail from Dr. Siegel's organization. For catalogs and information, write to: Exceptional Cancer Patients, 1302 Chapel Street, New Haven, CT 06511.)

I started another journal to record Ray's reactions to these new visual journeys. In the first tape, I took him on a journey through his body, as the book suggested, to specific places in his abdomen where healing was needed. Then I brought him to a house which had an immune and circulation room. The house image was symbolic of the body, and in this room Ray was given instructions of things to do in reference to his immune system.

Amazingly, when he got to the part where he requested to see his guide, he met a beautiful young woman with long brown hair. She was straight and tall and wore a long purple dress. Yellow flowers were pinned to her left shoulder. He told me he could not see her face clearly but communicated telepathically with her. Although she didn't say much, he knew that she wanted to show him things. He found himself in a beautiful garden full of vividly colored flowers. Then they walked to a great cliff overlooking the ocean. It was all very beautiful. He felt she was showing him all of this because even though this beauty was always around him, he never really took the time to appreciate it.

When Ray had my voice guiding him along, telling him what he would see and what he was supposed to do, it became very easy for him. In subsequent tapes I varied the journeys to different places, and either incorporated many scenes or just a few. The message at the end of the tapes always suggested that he meet his guide, in order to ask questions and receive answers. It was the only part of the tape where I didn't guide the journey. Ray had instant benefits from the first tape and would always meet his guide before his inner journey ended.

I changed the second tape somewhat, reenforcing the section where he stopped to work on his immune system. I added the following:

> "In the immune circulation room, there is a button and switch. Look and find the button marked 'Stop confused cell growth.' Push the button hard. Look and find the switch marked 'Normal healthy functioning cells,' and pull the switch to ON [this was repeated twice]; the healthy functioning cells know for certain what their job is now."

After Ray used the tape that contained the changes, he related to me that when he checked out his body, he found disease in the chest cavity and abdomen, and growths around the colon. The tumors, he said, looked like pieces of rotten sausage. He went into a room and pushed the STOP button for confused cell growth. Then he pulled the proper normal healthy switch and saw it was connected to a network of pipes and wires.

The visualizations on this tape were quite extensive. (I only related a small part of what they contained.) But we were beginning to realize the value of Dr. Siegel's work and how using these tapes could be applied to any disease. The results, after adding reenforcement on the second playing, were also quite beneficial in freeing Ray from pain. The experience gave him a feeling of well-being because he felt that he was now playing an active part in his own healing. It was somewhat different from his meditations, where either the visual aspects would come to him without conscious control or he was only able to zap the tumors with light. Not that what he had been doing all along wasn't wonderful, but these new tapes actually piloted him there, allowing him to see himself as his own healer and control his disease from the immune room.

In one of these taped guided meditations, I suggested he find a treasure chest along the path, open it, and look inside to see if there was a message for him. He told me he had found the chest. When he opened it, the message inside said, "Don't give up. Have faith and hope."

As he used the tapes, Ray continued to meet his guide. He told me he asked her name and she told him, "Christina." She soon began to help him directly in remarkable ways within his meditations. Here's an especially vivid one, just as I wrote it down.

"We were standing along the path," Ray said, "and I told Christina I wanted to know more about my sickness."

"You have a heavy sickness," she said.

Then he asked her what he could do to help himself.

"Maintain your faith and hope," she said, "and I will be available to help you."

He followed her and she led him this time onto a path to the left, where he saw the same scenery he had seen last time. This path, as well as the prior path, led to the same place—the top of the cliff. He asked her again, "What can I do to help myself?"

She was now behind him and put her hand on his right shoulder and said, "You must eat more of everything." He then started to leave and she asked him, "What are you going to do?"

"I'm going to go down to the beach and fly with the sea gulls," he said.

She had a small smile on her face and said, "Sea gulls fly, and you'll be floating."

Then he left and went to the beach.

Each time he met Christina he told me the color of her dress, while I tried to equate the significance of the colors. However, I hadn't a clue. She always had the same dress on, but it was of a different color. The flowers pinned to her left shoulder also changed in color. I guess I never questioned the appearance of Christina. I knew that his higher self was helping him, and I never questioned the how of it. I assumed Christina was a guide or his guardian angel manifesting in a form to which he could relate. It really didn't matter. He could speak with her and ask her questions, and he felt that she had great wisdom. He never wondered who she was, either. She just appeared and that was that. I noted that the phraseology of Christina's messages were not as Ray would have expressed them himself.

In another journey he asked Christina for a miracle.

She said, "There is a right time and a wrong time for a miracle. A miracle is God's will. You are an impatient man; patience goes with faith and hope."

This particular time she wore a silver blue dress and a white orchid on her shoulder. She told him that she would help him obtain a miracle.

I continued to feel that Ray would find his miracle, but more and more I felt that it might not be what he had in mind. I was grateful that he had already received so many miracles. After all, he had experienced numerous conscious encounters with his higher self, a dramatic out-of-body experience, and meditations that he had achieved on his own in which he had been able to diagnose his own body. He'd learned to use color to treat his tumors and to actually see the results. Our use of Reiki, TRT, and prayer communion had freed him from pain. He'd received dreams that contained informative messages, and now he was speaking lucidly with a wise and kindly guide who had become a great comfort to him. And, wonder of wonders, despite the fact that Christina was not "real," Ray accepted his encounters with her as being perfectly natural. I thought about the logical engineer I knew and what he would have said ten years before, if others told him they had met their "guide." However, I was overjoyed for him and told him more than once, "You've come a long way, baby!" He would always laugh when I said that.

One of his most beautiful encounters with Christina came a short time later. I didn't understand it at first.

Ray found a message in his treasure chest that said, "You are an exceptional soldier, but the battle has just begun." Then he met Christina and told her about it.

She said, "What have I been telling you which will be key for this battle?"

Ray asked, "Have faith?"

"No," said Christina. "That's not what I emphasized; I emphasized to have *patience*. Exceptional soldiers do not have patience. They wish to win today. But this battle is not like that. It's going to take longer, but faith will prevail."

This message indicated to me that *patience* was one of the lessons that Ray was struggling with in this lifetime. I sensed that his need for patience was strongly tied into the cause of his illness and that his illness had afforded him the conditions in which to make great strides in that lesson. I remembered that Edgar Cayce had said that patience is the chief cornerstone of soul development.

Ray and I both felt that he was advancing on his spiritual path. Actually having this sense of forward motion was new and stimulating for him. He was reaching into a part of himself that had been previously unknown to him consciously, though it had always been vaguely familiar. It gave him a great sense of peace while providing him the tools to relieve his physical discomfort. To help this continue, I wanted to further modify the tape for his needs. So I made the suggestions stronger on subsequent tapes to fight the invading cancer cells. It was our hope that the tapes would give him some relief from the constant nausea caused by his last chemotherapy treatment which was preventing him from eating anything substantial.

As I recall those days of June 1986, time seemed to stand

still. At the same moment, it was rushing right over me. I wanted it to move faster, yet I was afraid that this was to be the last of our days together. Time itself seemed to be alive: manipulating us, ceaselessly pressing us forward into good and bad moments, forcing me to prepare myself as if he were getting ready to leave me—although I had no idea how to do that. I prayed for time to move on "fast forward," when my faith would come alive again, to the time of our expected miracle. But how would I prepare myself if the miracle we received didn't actually spare his life?

I was beginning to feel the presence of the darkness that was wearing the gigantic cloak hooding us all, but I was afraid to look under that cloak. I knew that the presence was fear; I knew that death was only a transformation; but I could not dispel my simple raw human fear.

At long last I realized that I could do nothing to change the chain of events that may have been put into motion an eternity ago from cumulative events in many lives—events that now needed balancing. I preferred the word "balance" rather than "karma." From my understanding of Edgar Cayce's views on reincarnation, souls accumulate the results of their actions, both good and bad, from lifetime to lifetime. The Law of Cause and Effect always brings them back into balance. A soul chooses the settings and circumstances where it will best be able to work out the needed balance each time it incarnates. Perhaps Ray was on a mission in this lifetime to balance old debts and learn lessons that I could never understand. Maybe this illness was the only way he could fulfill the neglected lessons of many previous lifetimes. Ultimately, I felt that I had no say in the outcome of the next few months. Whatever was to happen, I could not change it.

Somehow a calmness was descending upon me. I found myself with new energy to help me cope with the day-to-day stress.

Ray and I continued with the taped visualization journeys

which alleviated some of his nauseousness. These new journey tapes involved him. He was able to ask Christina questions, go into rooms, press control buttons, and he was freed from pain. I felt that he was becoming more attuned to the spiritual side of himself and that Christina, whoever she was, was giving him great comfort.

Dr. Thomas called shortly after and told us he was "not too displeased" with the new lab work that had just come in. However, he reported that, although the count wasn't "too bad," there were some cancer cells in the fluid they took from his lungs. I thought to myself, what is the difference between too bad, a little bad, and bad bad? It was still cancer cells in the lungs. I recalled that, after using the first journey tape, Ray reported disease in the chest cavity when he scanned his body for sickness. He told me this over two weeks before.

I had read in Dr. Siegel's book about the art therapy work that he was doing with his patients and wanted to know more about it. I called Dr. Siegel's center in Connecticut; they promised to send the papers for Ray to do the drawings. When I returned the finished drawings to them, I was told that they would evaluate them and give us a report.

We kept going in every direction possible in June; sometimes I wondered why I continued to reach out for alternative ideas. I pondered that one day and realized that every alternative method seemed to come into our lives when Ray was ready for it. Maybe that was the way it was supposed to be.

Ray's weight was down to 125, and his spirits were dwindling with it. Our financial situation was also sliding downhill. He had to make the decision to go on disability, which didn't help his depression—especially knowing that he could no longer work. There would be no more paychecks coming in. I couldn't leave him alone in the house, so I couldn't work either. I also wanted to be with him if this was to be the last of our time together. The insurance was paying most of the medical bills, but there were plenty more bills for us to take care of. Whatever savings we had began to drain away.

A few days later Ray told me that he had worked a long time that morning in meditation. After first checking over his body, he said he actually saw what was in there. He didn't feel he was making any headway, but when he continued on his visualized journey, he met Christina. He told her that he wanted to get rid of all his diseased cells. He said she told him, "Be patient. It took years of stress to make them, and it will take awhile to undo."

Ray used the tapes every morning; sometimes in the middle of the day and again at night. Each time he meditated now he would pass a road sign on which was painted the message *Don't give up*. After another taped journey he told me he found in the treasure chest some blue books on faith. One was marked *The Book of Faith—6 Books,* and it was on top. When he met Christina, she had on her white dress with a red flower that looked like an opened rose. There were six paths that diverged out, all ending in the same place. She pointed to the path on the right, and Ray came up on the cliffs again. We weren't certain what the paths represented.

On the tape, I had suggested that he could fly through the air and carry three items with him to dispel into the air. He told me he dispelled three important aspects of his illness.

The next day we had an appointment with Dr. Thomas. Ray told me he just couldn't make it. I called the doctor and said that Ray was too weak. Dr. Thomas simply said to "Let it go."

Unlike the previous chemo medicine, the Platinol didn't come with "rescue pills" to stave off its ill effects on bone marrow. Ray just couldn't seem to recover from the side effects of the Platinol. Dr. Thomas never said to Ray, "You have to take it." He left it up to him to decide after he had spelled everything out. I was of the opinion that the drug would kill him. But I knew it was not up to me to tell Ray that he could not have what he believed to be his last medical hope. Ray just said, "I need to take the medicine."

I had to prevail over my fears and go along with Ray because I had no other choice. I recalled my beautiful cosmic dream more often now and tried to draw sustenance from it. I was feeling a strange dichotomy within me, almost like a separation within myself. The anxiety was from my emotional human side, but deeper within I felt a calmer "knowing" feeling. Yet I couldn't seem to gain access to it, however hard I tried. I could function only in that constant emotional anxiety. Of course, the girls were visiting on and off, but I was alone with Ray most of the time. When I looked at myself in the mirror, I didn't like what I saw.

After much deliberation with myself and discussion with Ray, we decided to ask Betsy to come back and live with us. We had a big five-bedroom house; there would be plenty of room. Asking her to move in was hard to do, because I didn't want to interfere with her life. But I had reached a point where I was becoming so stressed that I was afraid to be by myself. Betsy agreed. We didn't anticipate any problems. The nights, which had seemed so interminable, would be a bit easier now.

Six months after Ray's diagnosis I felt that he had actually left us a long time before. But I wondered why I would think such a silly thing because he was still with us. The cancer was relentless, continuing on and on with tenacity. I wondered how much more he could endure. I didn't want him to leave, but that was also selfish of me. I walked a gray line of not knowing how I truly felt, wanting him to stay with me, yet seeing how much he suffered. I wished it were over, if there was no chance that he would get better.

When the art therapy material from the Exceptional Cancer Patient Center came, Ray wanted to get right to it. At that time the Center used art therapy extensively, and I was anxious to learn more about it when we attended Dr. Siegel's June 20th seminar in Allentown. Ray sat in bed and, as instructed, drew pictures of the suggested subjects. My heart hurt so badly as I watched him, imagining him as a small boy with his crayons, coloring carefully. There was something of a dreamlike, unreal quality about the whole scene I was watching. A feeling came over me that this just couldn't be happening. An image jelled in my head of Ray, confidently standing before hundreds of top business executives, leading a seminar—and that was only a year before. The next day was Father's Day, and I was determined to get him out of bed for awhile.

Father's Day turned into an excellent day, providing us with some much-needed joy. Ray managed to come downstairs for most of the afternoon while we were all together. His mother was there with us, too. Gina called from Ireland, and Ray enjoyed their talk. His mom gave him a crocheted lap robe; Cindy surprised him with a very sophisticated short-wave radio so he could listen to all the foreign stations. Betsy presented him with two beautiful pictures: one of a beach scene and another of an airplane. He was most happy with the airplane picture and told her he would hang the pictures up tomorrow near his bed. Holly gave him an intercom, which was greatly appreciated. Luke made him an apple pie in school. We all oh'd and ah'd over it—much to Luke's delight, as noted by the big grin on his face. The other little ones gave him clothes, as I did. The afternoon was grand; we hated to see it end. Soon after, Ray started to gain ground; his appetite increased and the food was staying down.

Annmarie had told me about Mary, a healer who worked with cancer patients in many of the large hospitals. She worked strictly behind the scenes there, but the doctors asked for her because she did wonders for very ill and terminal cancer patients. Allievating fear and discomfort was her forte. She had the ability to tune in to the emotions of another and get right into the patient's psyche. I told Ray about her and asked him if he would like to see her. We were fortunate because she told me she would be able to visit us the next day.

We found Mary to be a lovely, calm person who exuded a

remarkable outward tranquillity, which she passed along to us in great quantity. I asked her how she tuned in on others. She told me she meditated along with the patient, and somehow was able to align and join the other's meditation. She sat with Ray silently for awhile, then remarkably asked him who the lovely young woman was. She then proceeded to describe Christina perfectly. Ray was quite surprised and inspired. Mary told him that he was very strong and fighting a big battle, that he had amazing healing powers and could have been a healer. She informed me later, when we were alone, that Ray had not made a definite choice one way or the other yet about his life.

On June 20, I made arrangements for my friend Liz to stay with Ray while I went to Allentown for Dr. Siegel's seminar. I found it deeply inspiring, soaking up his advice and concepts like a sponge. Dr. Siegel was vibrant, energetic, and positive in his beliefs. His own energy vibrated through the audience and filled the room. He was the first medical doctor that I knew of who lectured publicly about the fact that emotions were an integral part of the cancer process. He stated how necessary it was for patients to be able to first express repressed anger, which symbolically had eaten away at them, and then understand it, which would allow them to rid themselves of it. He felt that therapy for such patients played a large part in their understanding and ability to come to grips with their repressed rage.

Dr. Siegel said it was a positive reaction for patients to express their anger at the cancer, then to try to understand through therapy more of their inner workings. I felt like standing up and cheering, because the truth of Dr. Siegel's statements had struck us all. I couldn't help wondering why therapy wasn't included immediately in any cancer patient's overall medical treatment. I also wondered if it was too late for Ray to get into therapy.

I taped the entire seminar so that I could play it for Ray.

After it was over, I spoke to Dr. Siegel about Ray and where he was in the course of his illness. I told him that we had sent his artwork to the Center. He kindly assured me that he would personally check Ray's drawings and call me.

Around that time we had a few bad days, emotionally. Ray was depressed and would not say more than a few words. I wondered if it had anything to do with what he had heard on Dr. Siegel's tapes. I stopped myself momentarily and had to remember the breakthroughs we had had the last few months in our intimate communications. Just because he didn't want to constantly communicate, was I going off the deep end again? I realized how I had been pushing him the last few days, out of my own need, and I decided to step back and leave him alone.

I found that physical activity was good for me, so I started to take long walks with the dog and kept busy doing chores that I had let go in the house. Betsy and Cindy tried to talk to their father, but they, too, were met with resistive silence. They must have gotten through eventually, however, because Ray later told me he would try not to withdraw from us again. It was so very hard for him.

I remember sitting on the side porch with him a few days later when he told me he had a dream in which Christina asked him if he thought "they" (meaning the doctors) had told him how seriously ill he was. The cells had invaded his lungs, even though the count wasn't high. Nevertheless, the invasion had been launched. Christina was telling him that it was extremely serious.

That night I asked the Holy Spirit to send me a message, telling me the outcome of Ray's illness. I fervently pleaded that I be shown what was going to happen. That night I received my answer. The next morning, I recorded the dream in detail. I had dreamed that Ray and I were running down a rocky, sandy road, which was sloped toward the sea. Ray had just escaped from a large prison with my help. I looked over to the right and there stood an enormous, medieval arabesque structure which had been his prison. It was made of sandstone or some sandy material and reminded me of a large sand castle that children build on the beach in summer. The day was bright and sunny. I was aware of a deep blue sky overhead.

I was terrified, and we ran very fast down to the water. We were afraid that we were being chased and of his being recaptured and returned to the prison. I could see bars on the windows of this beautiful, seemingly benign palace. As we approached the water, I realized that it was not an ocean as I had first thought, but a river. I could see papyrus reeds growing near the shore, and I knew without a doubt that it was the river Styx.

Anchored in the reeds was a wooden boat, almost like a dugout, but with a bow, rising both in the front and the back. We quickly got into the boat and started paddling out onto the river. It wasn't quite twilight now, and the sun was starting to set, bright orange on the horizon. We could see clearly as the dimming twilight seemed to etch shapes and sharp contours on the water against the soft fading light. I was happily anticipating crossing the river now, getting far away from the prison. I thought it odd that no one was chasing us, but I knew we had to cross over to be safe.

The sun was a bright orange-red ball, lowering itself below the horizon and leaving a rippled path of color like a road— wide and shiny at its point under the earth's rim and then narrowing down to a small path by our boat. We were in the middle of the river, crossing into safety, when I turned around to see Ray, who was leaning out over the side of the boat. Then swiftly and silently he slipped under the water. I was stunned. It had happened so quickly and deliberately, I didn't have time to stop him. I couldn't imagine why he had done such a thing when freedom was only a short distance away.

I awakened with a start. At that point I was still very much in the dream. I lay quietly without moving and tried to analyze my dream. After I ran through it again, I knew then that Ray had made his choice. I decided to also send this dream to Mr. Irion at the A.R.E. for help in interpreting it.

When Ray would be leaving, I didn't know, but I wouldn't speak to him of my dream. I didn't really have to. His soul knew what I had just been shown. I decided to go along with whatever he wanted. It was hands-off time for me now, an extremely difficult situation.

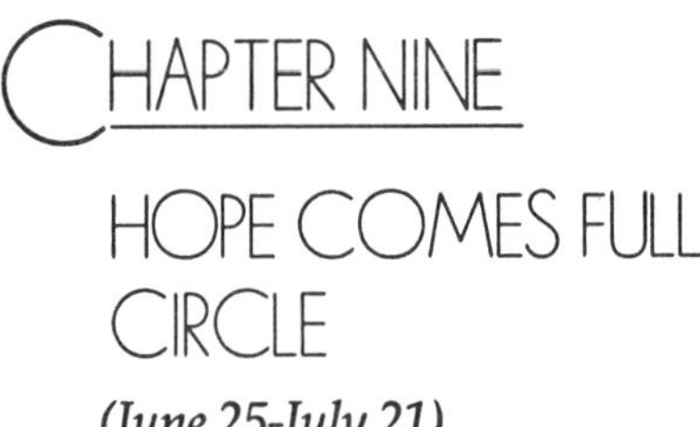

Chapter Nine

Hope Comes Full Circle

(June 25-July 21)

Early one morning in the beginning of June, Gina called from overseas. Before she spoke to Ray, she asked me if she should come home. Evidently Ray knew what she was asking, took the phone from me, and told her he was fine. "Let her enjoy herself," he said to me after he hung up.

Later that morning we saw Dr. Thomas and were relieved when he gave us a good report. He felt the tumors had shrunk and softened some and that the new chemo was working. He took blood for a workup and sent a sample to the Princeton lab so they could establish a new cancer count. Nothing would be decided about the next chemo until the reports came back. Ray felt good about the positive news and he vowed to get back at least a few of the pounds he had lost.

Mary and Annmarie were waiting for us when we arrived home. Mary went upstairs with Ray to sit and meditate with him, while I visited with Annmarie. Mary told me later that Ray was continuing to fight, but she felt he was still in the midst of soul decision-making. She didn't say any more. I had to remember that what Mary did was very personal. She actually joined Ray mentally when he meditated. Mary always informed the patient about what she was going to do and asked permission. After she finished, Ray was feeling good, and he told me how much he enjoyed "drifting" off with her.

In the afternoon Bernie Siegel called to discuss Ray's drawings. Right away he asked me to call him Bernie. He was such a busy man, and I appreciated his call. Ray was sleeping, and Bernie told me not to wake him up. After I spoke to him for a few minutes, I found it amazing that he had gleaned so much information from the three drawings that Ray had done. There were positive and negative aspects that he had seen in the drawings. Dr. Siegel's interpretation of the drawings revealed that Ray did feel intellectually that the chemo drug was good for him, but he was not taking it in or accepting it completely from an emotional level.

Ray had been asked to draw a picture of himself while he was receiving his chemotherapy treatment. A yellow bottle he had drawn with the drug in it connected to the exterior of his body, but did not go inside. He had not drawn hands or feet on himself. Bernie felt that this meant that Ray had no real control or grasp of the situation. The small head Ray had portrayed on himself was good, meaning that there was no intellectualizing of the illness itself.

The second picture Ray had drawn showed a path which represented the intestines. Bernie liked this one. He told me it was very colorful, the page was full, and Ray had drawn six white circles with flowers. The colors were good, but he wanted to know what the flowers were. After I explained that Ray was in his visualized garden where he sent himself during meditation, Bernie concluded that the tapes and meditations were working well. At that point, Ray woke up and joined us on the phone. Bernie asked him which way he was going on his path, and Ray said, "Up."

Ray had used arrows to denote white cells destroying the cancer cells. Bernie said this was not strong enough; we were to use pigs or sharks or something aggressive, yet of Ray's choosing. Bernie also wanted the nourishment to the tumors to be turned off much more aggressively. The third drawing of the house and family was not very positive. It showed Ray's outward lack of communication with his daughters, which seemed to be an overwhelming problem to him. I did tell Bernie that Ray and I and the girls were aware of this and asked him what he suggested Ray do about it.

Dr. Siegel advised us to get into some kind of therapy group that was familiar with his methods. He said Connecticut was too far for Ray to travel in his present condition, so he gave us the name of a therapist in Princeton, New Jersey—about an hour's drive for us. The therapist had just completed her training in Dr. Siegel's methods, and he spoke very highly of her.

Later that night, Ray meditated and told me that Christina suggested he use orca whales to represent his white cells. Wonderful! What could be more aggressive but still beautiful than orcas? I noted an interesting characteristic of the species—orcas are the only whales with teeth!

I meditated that night with the thought of the orcas and asked for a dream that would reveal any further information I should use in a new tape for Ray. I didn't remember any dream that night, but the next morning I made Ray a tape and the content of it surprised me. Perhaps I had dreamed about it after all. I had focused in on images of orca whales destroying the cancer cells, and the words streamed forth, coming quickly as I wrote them down to prepare his new tape. I recorded it and Ray said he loved it, that it felt right. I had him visualize highly aggressive orcas destroying the cancer cells. He easily associated with the suggested images.

Ray always felt good after this tape and never tired of it. He would describe the activity to me; he would actually be there with the orcas. Christina was there, too, on each journey, although he did not speak with her every time. The orcas came to be a symbol to him of his active participation in his illness, and the huge whales became a part of it to all of us. The girls would ask him how his orcas were doing, and he would laugh. We were surprised how intimately integral these white orcas became in all our lives. It was as though Christina had given them to us as a gift.

Toward the middle of June, Ray was eating better and had gained five pounds. He continued to listen to the orca tape untiringly. I had made other tapes for him, but I felt that the orca tape was the most aggressive and important one to date. He was able to conjure up marvelous and forceful imagery from it.

Ray continued to improve. Within ten days he had gained seven pounds. I found this amazing and prayed that it would continue, but I could never dispel what my inner self knew. His pain and the rigidity of his abdomen were subsiding, and the tape did relieve discomfort for extended periods of time. He had been able to reduce his pain medication considerably.

Betsy's move was finally completed, but we had a real mess to sort out. Life's course seldom runs smoothly. Luke tripped and cut his head on the coffee table, so Betsy made a run to the emergency room for stitches. He was not seriously hurt, but it frightened us all.

Ray's attitude and physical condition continued to improve. I started questioning everything again and was so uncertain now about the outcome. What made me think that my instincts and psychic insights were absolute? My eyes were seeing definite improvements in Ray's health, but my inner self was calmly resolute because that part of me had already received an answer. It was a horrendous spot to be in; I wasn't sure if I should trust my eyes or my inner self's messages. I couldn't release the images in my dream of the river Styx, and I didn't have positive inner feelings that he was going to make it.

Nancy, the therapist whom Dr. Siegel recommended, called,

and we set up an appointment for July 7. She asked me not to tell her anything about Ray so that she would have no preconceptions. She was going to Connecticut before she saw us and would pick up Ray's drawings to study them. She requested that the whole family join in that first session. Even Gina was to visualize herself with us and via a letter was to send along any comments that she wanted to contribute.

The end of June brought beautiful weather. Ray enjoyed getting out in the car again. Shortly after, we stopped at Dr. Thomas' office to pick up a prescription. Ray told him about the seven pounds that he had gained. They were both very pleased. The doctor said that his blood counts were all good and he could get on with the next chemo treatment. I didn't say anything. I didn't even want to talk about the new drug. I feared that if he had another treatment it would finish him.

July 4 was a grand day. We barbecued out in the back yard. Ray felt good and joined us all day and ate well. His stomach was softening more, and the pain was less. I sat and thought what our lives would be like by the next 4th of July. Sometimes I thought I was a masochist and couldn't enjoy any positiveness at all. I was an open wound, living daily in vulnerability. I had no recourse. There was no way to protect myself emotionally. By July 7 we were in the middle of a heat wave. The 90-degree weather wilted and frazzled us. For our appointment with Nancy we drove across the river to New Jersey with the air conditioner on high blast.

Nancy was in her early forties, tall and slim with dark hair. She was very personable and attentive in listening to us. She had a great deal of savvy, and we all liked her.

Nancy had a different approach, acting more as a friend, with none of the authority that "professional" counselors so often assume. I felt that she would be able to help Ray and, as the result of helping him, we would all benefit. The hour-and-a-half session was over too soon. Ray commented how much he had enjoyed Nancy. That first meeting was more of an orientation for Nancy to become familiar with us, as she tried to weave each of our personalities into the family situation.

One night shortly after, I dreamed that Ray had died and that my deceased father came to help me with the arrangements. In the dream I had not been with Ray when he died and that upset me dreadfully because I was also being told how important it was to be with him. I didn't know until that moment in my dream how terrible the grief could be. Then suddenly in the dream there was a flash of a woman who had handled a similar situation so calmly and serenely. I wished that I could do it like she had. I tucked this bit of information away in my mind.

Evidently, I was also being told through my dreams, over and over, that I should prepare myself for what was going to happen. But how does one prepare oneself for something like this? I felt as though the dark cloak of fear was wrapping tighter around me, and I could not maneuver out of the shadows of my own feelings of foreboding. Even though I saw that Ray was doing better physically, my state of mind was becoming more anxious. I could not sleep, and I was nauseated and panicky all the time.

There is an entry in my journal for July 10 which reads, "Ray was supposed to call Dr. Siegel today, but he said he wasn't up to it. I won't push him. He will do what he wants to do." I recall that day because I couldn't understand why he didn't want to take the initiative to call. Then it struck me. Was his work with Dr. Siegel reminding him of the psychotherapy he'd tried years before? I wondered if this had anything to do with the soul decision he had made—the one that had been revealed in my dream of the river Styx. Whatever the reason, I again felt helpless to do anything about it.

The next morning we went to see Dr. Thomas. I really didn't want to go with Ray because I knew we would have to discuss the upcoming chemotherapy treatment. I dreaded even talking about it. I told Ray again on the drive over that I thought the drug was disastrous, but he reminded me how well he had been doing since the last treatment. I gave up, and we drove the rest of the way in silence.

The doctor remarked that Ray looked rather pale, so he wanted to do a red-blood cell count to see if he would need a transfusion before the treatment. They continued to discuss it, and I remained silent. The doctor told him that they would administer the medication in a smaller dose this time. He was very pleased with Ray's positive weight gain; however, the most recent cancer count was not yet back from the lab. Ray's lungs and chest were clear, so the doctor said he saw no reason, if Ray was agreeable, to go ahead with the chemo on July 22. I swallowed hard and said nothing. I wondered if my psyche would survive until the 22nd of July. I had been with Ray twenty-four hours a day for the last six months, an emotional participant in this awful kidnapping.

The scheduling of the second chemotherapy had completely undone me. I couldn't handle this knowledge nor the fright that ensued when I thought about it. I felt ashamed, because Ray was the one suffering so terribly. But something was suddenly telling me to remove myself physically, if only for a few days.

Then a foreign thought popped into my head, about really getting away for a few days. I thought about visiting my friend, Norella, in Florida, sitting in the sun, away from the sickness, where I could try to regain some emotional strength and balancing. It seemed like a bizarre thought at first, to leave for a few days. I laid awake that night thinking about why I would want to do such a thing and why the thought had popped so abruptly into my head. I tried to look at it objectively. I realized suddenly and with clarity that I had become consumed by Ray's illness and his journey. Instead of my being a helping partner, I had allowed myself to be completely crushed by it. It wasn't my journey; it was his. I was losing myself in him and that was not being helpful to him.

It was hard to explain, but from the moment the thought of a trip came to me, I knew it would manifest, even before I had made the conscious decision to go. I had to do it. There was some important reason why I had to detach myself for a short time. It only came to my mind much later that Florida had been my balancing place once before. I told Ray that I would like to get away for a long weekend, and he encouraged me to go. He reminded me that I would be gone for only a few days. I didn't tell him everything that I had been thinking because I felt it was just for me. Betsy was there, and the other girls were in and out and could look after him. The girls also told me to go.

Something in my inner self had already decided I would go. Of course, I would be back in time for the chemo. Ray kept repeating that there were plenty of people around to take care of him. However, I questioned whether they could care for him as well as I did and if he could get along without me. We had not discussed the next treatment. I knew that he would go on with it, and I needed all the courage I could muster to help him get through it.

Mary came that afternoon to sit and meditate with Ray. She felt he was doing good work in the tumor area, and together they visualized an enormous amount of energy to bolster Ray's weakened body. Ray laughed and told me that he actually felt the heat that he and Mary had generated visually together.

Mary got ready to leave and went out to her car. Two minutes later, however, she was back inside holding up her car keys. When she had taken the keys out of her pocket, she discovered that two of them were bent. She couldn't get the key into her ignition, so we had to straighten the two out with plyers before she could start her car. She remarked with a straight face, "I told you we generated a lot of energy." It was the only answer to how the keys had gotten bent in the first place. Mary had arrived in her car, gone up to sit with Ray, then came back down, and out to her car. But we were all living in a place where nothing surprised us any more.

Around the 13th of the month, I received a long, helpful letter from Mr. Irion at the A.R.E. in response to my request for his help in deciphering a number of my dreams. He was very kind and wrote me an extensive letter with his interpretations. My letter had reached his office while he was away on speaking engagements.

While employed at the A.R.E., Mr. Irion had spent many years researching the Edgar Cayce readings. He was the author of two books, *Interpreting The Revelation with Edgar Cayce* and *Vibrations* (both published by A.R.E. Press). He was also a frequent lecturer on the Revelation of St. John and on the subjects of dreams and vibrations. For over fifteen years he had conducted a weekly study group in Virginia Beach, Virginia, on the Book of the Revelation. Mr. Irion also wrote a column called "An Interpreter's Journal" for A.R.E.'s membership magazine, *Venture Inward*, which reported on and answered questions about dreams. It was always the first article I read in that marvelous magazine and was where I had first learned Mr. Irion's name.

I had sent him my serpent dream of last August, the one I felt had been chasing me all through Ray's illness. I don't think I had been ready until then to face an understanding of my nightmare. Here is that dream:

I was with two other people. One was Ray, the other was a younger person who was somehow familiar to me. This third person disappeared somewhere along in the dream. We were in the Tampa, St. Petersburg area of Florida, where we had lived for two of our seven years there. I knew that a violent hurricane was happening nearby, but it was calm where we were. In my dream, I wondered why we were there. We had lived in that area over twenty years ago.

Then we were in the car looking for a house to buy. Again, I wondered why we were looking in that particular area. We went under a bridge. I had the distinct impression that the entire countryside was of a lower elevation. Exactly on the other side of the bridge or overpass was another area familiar to me. Now we were in Pennsylvania. We came upon a large brick house, which was blindingly white and stood out against the drab landscape and low rolling hills. It was an old house that someone seemed to be fixing up. There was no "For Sale" sign on it, but I knew it was vacant.

The house was large and set up almost to the road. There was a storm ditch that separated the front yard from the road, and a wooden plank crossed over this ditch. You had to walk over the plank to get into the front yard, then up to the front door. The main part of the white house loomed above us, and an attachment, added to the right side, made it larger still. Ray and I got out to look. As we did so, I thought this would be an easy house for anyone to find as it was the first one sitting directly to the right and slightly under the overpass. Where the house sat in relationship to the overpass was extremely important to me.

Then I thought that that really wasn't a good enough reason to buy a house. For whatever explanation, it was urgent that it be easy to find and easy to give directions to it. We went into the front yard, then walked around to look at the back. There was a large stream running through the back yard, which opened into a smaller stream up a ways and to the right. The larger stream was shallow, very dirty, with logs and bits of floating debris. I had the impression there were even more bridges and piers of wood than I could see. Crossing and criss-crossing channels were everywhere.

In the back yard was a small pier. It stood at the junction where the larger and smaller streams joined. Ray and I stood on this main pier. At that moment as I looked at him, Ray was a young man. Suddenly without saying a word or giving any kind of warning, he decided to cross the stream or look for something. I couldn't imagine why he went down the small ladder hooked onto the pier that went into the water, but it was shallow, about knee high, so I wasn't worried. It did bother me, though, not knowing what he was doing.

He was near the pier after just entering the water, when I saw something moving off to my right, churning the water in the smaller offshoot channel and moving swiftly into the larger channel. It was gliding just under the surface, pushing the water above it into large swells, shooting ripples off to the side banks. I looked with horror at a gigantic snake moving toward us. It was monstrous. I screamed at Ray to hurry back out of the water onto the pier.

The huge serpent swam closer. Now I could see its large triangular-shaped head and shiny black eyes. It came right up to the dock and, raising its gross head, looked directly at me. The shiny black shoebutton eyes held mine. I was amazed to see an intelligence coming out, rather than the flat, black eyes of a reptile. The snake's gaze locked into mine and held me frozen where I stood, unable to break free of its almost mesmerizing force. The powerful creature looked like a giant anaconda.

Incredibly, I realized that I was not frightened by the snake. Of course, I didn't intend to go into the water with it, but I was not afraid of the snake itself, only of what it would do to Ray. I screamed repeatedly to him to hurry onto the pier, but he deliberately took his time. Terror overwhelmed me. I could not understand why he would not hurry. At last, he was climbing up the ladder onto the dock. One leg, from the knee down, was still in the water, however, when suddenly the snake reared straight up from the water and grabbed him around the knees and feet. I could see the snake's eyes clearly and its long, brownish body.

Terrified, I watched from my perch on the pier as this huge snake transformed itself into a gargantuan octopus with a giant hump and many short powerful tentacles. The monstrous creature from the dark underwater murk wrapped its tentacles around Ray, covered him with its huge humped body, and dragged him under the water. Ray's face was devoid of expression. He uttered no cry, nor did he attempt any struggle.

I screamed and shouted, hoping that the octopus would be distracted by the noise, but it didn't work. I watched with horror as this awful creature dragged him under. I saw bubbles coming up to the surface. Finally I was able to move. The words, "Get help, get help," shrieked through my head. I started to run to find someone, but stopped. There wasn't enough time. He could only be underwater a short time, and it seemed he was under such a long time already; perhaps he was dead by now. I really couldn't imagine how he could survive this terrible attack.

Hesitating a few more seconds, I knew that time had run out. There was no more waiting. The water was shallow, and I couldn't see any thrashing. So I jumped in to pull him out, praying that the octopus was gone. I was terribly frightened but knew I had to try. Feeling around in the water and not finding him only added to my unbearable anxiety. The phrase, "Do I have any more time?" repeatedly ran through my head. Walking back and forth, searching under the water, I found him at last and tried to pull him out. The octopus was gone. I thought that surely Ray had to be dead. Why else would the creature leave? Somehow, I managed to get him out and onto the pier.

The sun was shining brilliantly now; I saw green trees and brightness all around me. We were in the middle of a beautiful clear, large lake, surrounded by tall green fir trees that grew along the shore. I had the impression of being in the far north, high up in the mountains. The water was a deep blue with the sun reflecting brightly off the ripples of the lake, making it one large shimmering body. How did we get to this serene mountain lake? It puzzled me. The floating wooden dock was directly in the middle of this lovely lake. At first I thought it was floating unattached in the water, but then I realized it was anchored from underneath. Staring down at Ray, I was surprised to discover that he now looked like a windup toy, much like a child's metal roly-poly man, and he was very small. His metal body was encased in a hard plastic-like covering. His shirt was bright red and below were royal blue pants. His face had the smile of a toylike caricature stamped on it. A black belt was painted on his middle. He reminded me of the fairy tale characters, Tweedle Dum and Tweedle Dee. It confused me when I saw him; how could he have gone into the water one way and come out another way?

Instinctively I turned him over to drain the water out of his mouth, but first it was necessary to peel all the hard, clear, shellac-like plastic off his face to get to him. The plastic resembled the birth caul of a newborn pup. I finally got it off, turned him on his side, and began to drain the water out. But squeezing and pumping him, trying to get more out, only sent the water to his head. To my amazement and utter frustration, the water, instead of coming out his mouth, was blowing up his head like a balloon. Incredibly—and this also confused me—he was now breathing. The dock had moved into a small shallow area surrounded by green plants and reeds. I grabbed a long, open reed and stuck it down his throat to serve as a breathing tube. To my further amazement it also pumped the water out and enabled him to breathe in air, serving as a dual passageway. I knew he was all right, but different; he was not a human being any more.

Mr. Irion commented that my dream was operating with the symbology of our spiritual lives. He told me that the two other people were the unconscious souls of myself and Ray. The fact that we were in Florida indicated to him where/when the cancer problem probably had its inception. I was amazed to hear him confirm what I had suspected for a long time. He said he felt that cancer is a manifestation of rebellion at the soul level, which appears in the flesh so that we can gain a perspective about our rebellion in spirit. What I had sensed before, that this lifetime was a lesson in spirit for Ray, was also what Mr. Irion had gleaned from the dream. He went on to tell me that the hurricane had portended the cancer. The "looking for a *house* to buy" symbolized that Ray and I were looking for our temple, the body, where you really live and worship. Going under a bridge indicated that something could possibly have been avoided somewhere in our lives.

He pointed out that the countryside was at a lower elevation (soulwise) in our lives. We both went under the bridge (symbolically and actually for Ray), meaning that we had chosen to work things out in the physical, because the bridge or overpass area was familiar to me. Then, we found the substantial brick house. This was a symbol of the body, and it was close to the roadway of life. The storm ditch and the wooden plank was where we both "walked the plank" into the front yard, relating to the "front" we put on in life.

Mr. Irion said that the main part of the house loomed above us both, the higher life. Then, Ray and I walked around the house and looked at the back, the unconscious yard of life. Mr. Irion felt that here we had moved into the body unconsciousness where we found the flow of life, the flow of water, the spiritual life of both of us. Here, he wrote, we saw all kinds of bridges, piers, with criss-crossing channels. All of these were related to body functions, Mr. Irion explained.

Our stand on the small pier represented our stance in life. The smaller stream joining the larger one was the life force going into the larger unconscious life. This was where Ray, as a young man, stepped into the spiritual body of life (the large stream), although it seemed "shallow." Mr. Irion remarked that it was then that I noticed the gigantic snake, which he said actually represented the spirit of wisdom (the oldest symbol of wisdom) and the saving factor in all our lives. The snake looked directly into my eyes, a recognition of me as a helpmate to Ray, Mr. Irion said, as well as to myself. He wrote that I could not break free of its "mesmerizing" forces (a good thing that happened to me) and I was not frightened by the snake. He was my friend!

The snake "reared up" from the water (the spirit) and grabbed Ray around the feet and knees (the feet symbolize understanding and the knees, bowing to a higher force). I saw the snake's eyes (the "I's" of the snake), and then the snake turned into a giant "octopus"—the two-edged sword. The octopus had powerful tentacles. Ray could not recognize that the snake (wisdom) was also the octopus, and he didn't struggle. The octopus then dragged Ray under the water. I couldn't get help but had to do something on my own, Mr. Irion told me. I got into the spirit of life, the water, and back onto the pier (back to earth). It was at this point in my dream that I had the courage to save my husband.

The sun (the light of life) was shining brilliantly (clear understanding at the soul level), and I noticed the vastness of the beautiful lake (of life). No wonder I was puzzled.

Ray, as a plastic-covered, toy-like creature, was a symbol of what we really are, for the real life is our dream life—not the flesh and body life. The caul was his psychic life. So, this dream was actually a short story of Ray's entire life made up in symbols. As I tried to drain the water out of Ray, it went to his head, the ego life. Ray was now breathing through a reed. Mr. Irion reminded me about how Moses had been hidden among the reeds: "The passageway to life—breath," he wrote. The flesh life is really the dream, he mentioned, so with the reed I had awakened both Ray and myself to our spiritual reality. I knew he was all right in one way (the spiritual life) but not in the human—this was a clear image of the transformation that takes place between flesh consciousness and spirit consciousness, between life and death.

I found the dream interpretation from Mr. Irion extremely interesting and accurate. He had been able to put into words some important observations that I had only sensed. The most helpful bit of information that came out of the interpretation confirmed for me that many of our soul choices had been made in Florida. Our paths had diverged there, and I was now certain that it had been the true beginning of Ray's illness.

Mr. Irion also interpreted my dream of the river Styx. He pointed out that the dream began with the statement that Ray had just escaped from a "sand castle—medieval arabesque in appearance," which to him was where—and when—Ray built the foundation for his problem. It indicated that a past-life situation, perhaps in the Middle East during the Middle Ages, had brought about the circumstances for which Ray chose a traumatic illness as a solution.

About my cosmic dream, Mr. Irion said it had been a beautiful experience, reminiscent of portions of the Book of Revelation. Everything was peaceful, and I had felt one with the All. My experience is also described in portions of The Revelation, in chapter twenty-one, for example, where there is no darkness; all is light, warmth, and serenity. It is a place of tremendous love, a knowing; for God is the light, and I was one who possessed that enlightened love. It truly was a remembering of where I had come from, which could not be put into words. I felt extremely privileged when he said that my description of that state is one of the best he had ever read. He also stated that my understanding of the experience should be treasured—not to be told too often to others who had never had such experiences, because they simply would not be able to understand, nor would they try. He said that "Experience is the only teacher. Treasure it, but live it for your husband."

I decided, when I sent that dream to Mr. Irion, that I did want to share it with others. He must have realized this because he published the dream in its entirety in the December 1986 issue of *Venture Inward*.

I was especially grateful for Mr. Irion's interpretation of my dreams at the time they arrived, because he confirmed much of what my inner self had been trying to tell me. It was a strange coincidence that the letter arrived a few days before I left for Florida—the very place where so many of our soul decisions had been made years before. I began to realize how well informed spirit had kept me throughout Ray's illness. The dream interpretations from Mr. Irion had been important—they had confirmed for me that spirit was indeed by my side, accompanying and supporting me all along.

That afternoon, Ray called Bernie Siegel's office. They scheduled him for an October 3 appointment at their Center in Connecticut. Ray definitely wanted to meet Dr. Siegel face to face. At that point, however, I knew in my heart that he would never get there. Ray continued to gain weight; two more pounds. His appetite was good, and his pain kept decreasing between the more frequent meditation tapes and the now infrequent medication.

I left for Florida the 16th of July; my return ticket was for the 20th. As I was able to push aside my guilt about leaving, I was starting to look forward to seeing my friend. I had longed to be able to get a good night's sleep, sit in the sun without feeling the responsibilities of changing dressings, fixing meals, and dealing with terrible sickness. After I arrived and settled myself in my friend's back yard, I sat in the warm sun and wondered how I had forgotten that the world continued on as usual. Not only was I in Florida, I was on Merritt Island, as Ray had seen in his dream. This prompted me to go over the merits of my life. I meditated about the chain of events that had led up to this point in our lives.

We had taken different paths once before in Florida in this lifetime. I felt perhaps that I had now returned there to reinforce my feelings as I had done through therapy during those seven years. It also confirmed for me that I must continue on the path of freedom and healing, no matter which direction Ray was going. I thought about my serpent dream and wondered if I had been able to interpret it last August or if Ray had gone for a checkup, would it have made any difference. At that point I realized why I had been directed back to Florida for these few precious days.

By the time my rest in the Florida sun was over, I had come to realize the true spiritual depth of Ray's journey in this life. As I look back, understanding the origins of his journey had been vital for me. I was sure spirit had played its part in making that happen. I felt stronger because of it, more able to cope with the days ahead that I would have to face. I had also retrieved my own identity from the web of Ray's illness. The result was that I felt better prepared to help him.

Ray, Betsy, Sarah, and Luke met me at the airport. I was shocked when I saw Ray there, too. Just being away from him for this short time gave me a perspective I had not had before. I swallowed back my tears and wondered where my husband had gone. He looked like an old man. His face was a chalky color, and he was thin and gaunt. He'd lost so much hair. In my mind I still saw him as he used to be, tall and strong; not this stranger disguised as my husband. I turned my face away a moment to compose myself. The nightmare started to descend upon me, and cold, stark reality stared at me once again.

Betsy had let Ray drive to the airport because she felt he could do it, and she hadn't had the heart to say no. I asked her to drive home, though, so Ray and I could talk. He seemed angry and expressed it often over trivial things on the drive back. Later, he told me that it wasn't me he was angry at—it was his whole life situation.

We went to the doctor the next day for a checkup because Ray had developed a cough while I was away and the pain in his abdomen had returned. The chemo was still scheduled for the 22nd, which was two days later. But Ray told the doctor that he was not up to it. Dr. Thomas said maybe next week if he was feeling better. The cancer count had come back from the lab in Princeton and showed very little change. Ray was losing his appetite again, along with a few more pounds, and he was thoroughly discouraged. He asked the doctor for something stronger for the pain.

I had not questioned him yet about how often he was using the tapes since I had left. The medication was not working, and the doctor decided to put him on a morphine elixir. Dr. Thomas told us that it was up to Ray now to tell him what he wanted to do. The plan had been to keep a constant level of the Platinol drug in his system, but now, if he put the treatment off, it would negate whatever good the drug had done. If this chemo was not done, he said, the next chemo would be like starting all over again. It just had not worked out as the doctor would have preferred. But it happened this way, and that was the way it was. Dr. Thomas told me that he was amazed that Ray was still here with us after what they had seen during the first surgery back in January. We went home, disappointed and silent. I didn't know what to say to Ray. The dark depression hung in the air between us on the ride back home.

Chapter Ten

Permission to Say Good-By

(July 22-August 9)

Cindy stopped by the house early one morning in late July. She looked worried.

"Are you all right?" I asked her.

She told me she was on her way to work and had the sudden feeling to turn around. She said she was inexplicably driven to tell her father that she loved him. I asked her why she thought it happened specifically on that day.

"I'm not sure," she replied. "But Dad said, 'Me, too.' "

Cindy had especially acute psychic abilities. She was able to observe the energy bodies of others. I noticed from remarks she made that this was easier to do when someone was physically ill or asleep. I only realized later how much I took for granted all my daughters' gifts and their ways of thinking. We had always discussed philosophical and religious subjects openly from the time they were young. I strongly feel that children need some religious direction, so we attended church together regularly. Later, they would have the freedom to do what they wished with the information they had received.

Strangely, I never had a problem dovetailing my metaphysical beliefs with my Catholicism. I perceived even rigid doctrines differently than most people and was able to sense their underlying meanings. Cindy and Gina were more naturally in tune with metaphysics and more inquisitive. Holly didn't become interested until she was older, while Betsy, the quiet one, just took it all in. From what I could tell she, too, was finding her truth in our ways of thinking. So, by the time their father got sick, the girls and I were all pretty much aligned with an overall metaphysical philosophy.

It was July 22 and no one had spoken about the cancelled chemo. I felt it would be a disaster, but I continued to hold to my belief that ultimately, when he returned to it, chemotherapy would be Ray's choice. The doctor had left it up to him.

Gina called that night from Northern Ireland and told us she would be home on August 1. We were coming into the last week of July; it was hot and muggy. Ray had started on the morphine elixir. It made him sick the first few times, but he was doing better now. It settled him, lessened the pain, and enabled him to eat a little. Mary visited Ray once a week, and he looked forward to their meditation experiences together. He journeyed inwardly with his orca tape as often as he could, and we gave him Reiki treatments whenever possible.

As the days rolled by, I realized that the time I had been able to spend by myself in Florida had emotionally fortified me more than I knew. The constant anxiety and panic that were with me before I left had quieted. I was experiencing a definite shift of feeling, with the anger and post-troubles starting to dissolve. The strange calmness that had been hiding beneath my emotions seemed to have mysteriously risen closer to the surface. It was almost as though the clarity and oneness I had experienced during my cosmic dream had, at least temporarily, dissipated the emotional cloak that was smothering me.

I felt perfectly in the moment that day, not troubled by the past or worried about the future; only the present had become important—the *now*. It was as though I could see the events of the past, stretching back into previous lifetimes, as being only snapshots along the line of that eternal *now*. I wished all could feel it, have that bird's-eye view perspective of spirit as they live their lives.

As this new realization unfolded, my entire philosophy of life seemed to enter my consciousness, coming to full flower within me. So many past events that had seemed important then appeared trivial to me now, although they had all given us the opportunity to grow. Perhaps Ray and I had consciously made a contract somewhere in the past or had forged one through karma. Either way, through free will we still had to live in the here and now.

Ray's illness was a stark reality. But from this perspective, knowing how Ray got there, any other way would have left undone what he had chosen to resolve, one way or another, in this lifetime. Spirit was helping me to accept the dramatic workings of the universe, allowing me to truly know my part in it. Over the past few months, I had seen Ray progress from an analytical, logical engineer to one who engineers his dreams and navigates visually into the interior of his body.

I felt confident that Ray's astonishing spiritual growth in this lifetime would be etched deeply into his own eternal now and be carried forward with him forever. I, at least, felt gratitude that I had helped him do it. At some level I was sure that he was still surprised at how easily he developed once he turned to the light. When he asked for help, his own spirit—the part of him that is the essence of the Holy Spirit—was there for him, helping him balance his mistakes, heal the hurt from his childhood, open his heart, communicate to his family, and show him the path back to God. He was no longer an observer, but a full participant.

After I returned from Florida, I noticed that Ray's consciousness was starting to shift. I was sensing a different feeling from him, a change of vibration when I entered his presence. I asked him what he was feeling inside. He admitted that he was furious with the cancer and kept asking it to leave. He told me again that he realized his priorities had been all wrong in life. I assured him that he had been a caring, loving father and husband and to remember the good times we'd had, how he had always been there for all of us. He seemed to be constantly going back over his life now, rethinking the way things should have been done. I thought about how far he had come in this life, how his opening to spirit in the last six months had increased his inner awareness. I could only imagine how far into his karmic past it reached. I sat and looked into his eyes; my realization of his spiritual progress overwhelmed me.

On July 25, Ray told me that he had met Christina in his inner journey that morning. She told him that his condition was better than he visualized. Ray took it to mean his physical condition, but I thought she might have been referring to his spiritual state. My thoughts had started to shift back to the chemo again. Dr. Thomas had left the decision up to Ray whether to continue. I focused constantly on it without relief, and my emotional stress started to return. I didn't want him to go through the agony again. At that moment, the chemo was causing me more distress than the thought of him dying. I could not understand why he was putting himself through it. Then I thought, maybe it was to hasten things. I had strong feelings that he wouldn't survive the violent reactions to the chemo this time. Perhaps he knew it—perhaps this was also entering into his decision.

Cindy and Cathy returned from a week's vacation on Cape Cod and brought Ray a beautiful black and white ceramic orca whale mounted on a piece of driftwood. Cindy told him she would paint it all white, and he could use it in his orca journey. He just smiled.

We were due to see Nancy, the therapist, again and I wanted to discuss the chemo with her. I was hoping that I would be able to explain my feelings about it. I knew that I would be unable to stay with Ray while it was being administered. Ray got right into his positive feelings about the upcoming chemo.

He was sure in his mind that he wanted to go ahead with it. I had to express what I felt about not wanting to be with him during the treatment, though I didn't want to say anything more about the medicine being poisonous to his body. My throat would close whenever I started to speak about my inability to be with him during that time. I felt myself constructing a circular, solid wall of protection around myself to ward off the thoughts of that dreadful chemo.

Nancy immediately addressed the problem, telling me that I shouldn't be present when the treatment was given, because my negativity would interfere with its intended effect. She continued on to say that not only would I undermine Ray's confidence in the therapy, I was so negative that it would be reflected in everything associated with the chemo. I wasn't exactly sure what that meant. But she added that, while this was my prerogative, what mattered was what Ray wanted and how he felt about it. Ray told me that it was all right if I wasn't there with him, that it was his decision to go ahead. I mentioned to Nancy that someone had to be with him, so I suggested that we get a nurse. Immediately, Cindy and Holly said that they wanted to stay with their father while the treatment was given. I questioned them, to make sure that they knew what was involved. However, they were still positive and reminded me that Betsy would be able to come by and help, too.

Two nights before the chemo, Annmarie, Mary, the girls, and I conducted a healing circle for Ray. We joined hands as Ray sat in the center. Annmarie led us in prayer and called for the light, asking us to visualize a great white healing light around Ray. She asked us to pray for him in all positive ways; I wasn't sure what I was praying for, but only that it would have the greatest possible benefit to him, whatever the outcome.

On July 29, Ray entered the hospital. His chemotherapy treatment was scheduled for the next day. His blood counts were up to requirements, but the doctor was concerned about his overall weakness. When I heard that, I thought I would have a panic attack on the spot. Ray turned to me and said, "I have no choice. I have to take another shot at it."

They would administer the treatment on the 30th of July. Although Gina was supposed to be coming home August 1, she ended up booking whatever was available and would be arriving at JFK at 3:15 p.m. on July 30. This required additional planning. I was incapable of driving alone the two-and-a-half hours to New York. The threat of the chemo was making me almost nonfunctional. I felt completely inept and devastated.

We decided that Cindy would go to the hospital at 9:00 a.m. and stay with Ray. She would leave at noon, pick me up, and we would drive to the airport together. Holly would come down to the hospital at noon and stay with her dad until we returned around 5:00 p.m. Since the last chemo, Betsy had been transferred to the same hospital, so she would be able to drop in throughout the day. We would telephone Holly at intervals from the road during that time span. No one was quite comfortable with the arrangement for those five hours, but it was the best we could do.

The telephone rang at daybreak. I heard Gina's voice and immediately thought that something was wrong. She was calling from Ireland to assure me that she was ready to board her flight. I hung up and mentally figured that if she could get through customs quickly, we could beat the horrendous Long Island business traffic coming home. I called the airline and explained the situation, asking them to expedite Gina through customs and baggage. They assured me they would take care of it and took down all the information. I got up and walked over to the window to look out at the world and murmured a silent prayer.

Ray called me around 8:00 a.m. He said his blood work was fine and that there was no fluid around his lungs. Dr. Thomas felt that Ray would tolerate the chemo well. They were giving him heavy sedation, so he wouldn't remember the violent vomiting and other reactions. I thought about how the doctors said that this particular chemo had been used beneficially on other patients without such horrid side effects. Why did Ray have to have such a bad reaction? Cindy stopped by the hospital at about 9:30 a.m. Ray was experiencing some nausea, but Dr. Thomas hoped this time the drug would be easier on him. She left the hospital at noon as planned and picked me up. We left for JFK, making the trip in two hours.

I had prayed that everything would go smoothly at the airport because it was extremely important that we get back to Ray without any delays, but it wasn't long before the first disaster struck. Gina's flight was twenty-five minutes late because of sudden lightning and heavy rain moving into the area. Cindy and I stood and watched from the airport window as the rain and wind swept across the runways and tarmac. We knew that Gina was above us, helplessly circling and circling.

I couldn't even drink a cup of tea because I felt as if my stomach was up in my throat. Then, the plane miraculously appeared out of a heavy bank of clouds and rain, touching down onto the runway. Our spirits lifted. I was weak with relief as we hurried down to customs to meet her.

After fifteen or twenty minutes, however, we still hadn't seen Gina. Passenger after passenger exited through the door during the next half hour. I suspected that the airline personnel had not followed through in expediting. I could do nothing but stand by the door, anxiously awaiting the first glimpse of her face, while Cindy went to the telephone to call Holly at the hospital. In a moment, she dashed back and reported disastrous news. Ray had become severely nauseous and totally disoriented. He didn't know where he was and kept asking Holly to get him out. Holly was extremely upset, alone and unable to help him. The nurses had been in and out, but there was nothing more they could do for him. His disorientation was frightening to Holly. Cindy told her to call Betsy. The two of us went crazy when we heard all this, but we couldn't do anything either except stand by the door and wait.

People continued to exit through the customs doors, some accompanied by airline personnel. Those being expedited were neither sick nor old people, but young teen-agers, a woman in a wheelchair, and a child. I stopped two of the airline personnel and tried to talk to them. They told me they couldn't handle it and wouldn't listen to me. I hurried over to the ticket counter and explained the situation again. They informed me that they had no record of the arrangements. At that point of disembarking, they could do nothing to help. Cindy and I had reached such a frenzied peak of anxiety that I thought we would explode. Then I tried to call the airline headquarters, but no one answered the phone. We were trapped and nearly hysterical.

Finally at 4:45 p.m.—one hour later—Gina came running through the customs doors, disheveled and frantic, one of the last to be cleared. I was in a rage but hadn't the time to go back to the airline counter and vent it. Gina told me they had called out over the loudspeaker names of people with special deplaning arrangements, but her name was not called. She explained the situation to them, but no one seemed to care and no one helped. We went back to the telephone to call the hospital before we left the airport.

The next report was not good either. Betsy was now with Holly, and we spoke to her. Dr. Thomas had actually discussed the topic of "coding" or "no coding" with her. Essentially, this forced us to choose whether we wanted everything possible done for Ray to a point. If a major organ failed, would we want them to continue working on him? When we heard this, we fell apart in a frenzy of anxiety, while Gina searched the area frantically for a baggage cart. There was none to be had and no available redcaps either to give us any help.

We joined forces to lug Gina's monstrous suitcases out of the airport building to the other end of the parking lot. We finally reached the car and jammed her large, heavy suitcases into the trunk and back seat. We jumped into the car, then Cindy raced out of the parking lot and onto the highway. An hour later we stopped again to call. Holly had another bad report—the drug was not being excreted properly through Ray's kidneys, and the doctor had to catheterize him to get the drug flowing. It was desperate news; Gina was frantic and Cindy was a nervous wreck as she drove. I sat and sobbed softly, terrified that my worst fears would be realized, that Ray would leave us before we arrived back at the hospital— and then we got stuck in rush-hour traffic.

We stopped and called again at 7:00 p.m., but the doctor had left because of another emergency. He said he would call the hospital at 8:30 p.m. Betsy and Holly were both with Ray, waiting for us, so we were off again, madly racing down the turnpike. I prayed to God and the Holy Spirit and sent messages to Ray not to leave us until we got there.

We finally arrived at 8:00 p.m. and rushed into his room. I cursed the airline personnel again and again. It had taken us three-and-a-half hours to drive back. Ray looked horrendous, but the worst was thankfully over and he was now sleeping. Dr. Thomas called the hospital at 8:30 p.m., as he had promised. He told me he was surprised that there was no fluid around Ray's lungs. He decided to put him on antibiotics anyway because he had developed another cough. He would see how Ray was the next day and decide then whether or not to release him.

Holly had been devastated by the events she had witnessed that day. Ray had kept asking her to get him out of the room; he even tried to pull out the tubes. I was so sorry that she had been alone with him, and I cursed myself for not insisting on a private nurse. She cried and said it had been horrible when she couldn't help him. Thank God, Betsy had been able to join her. She said if she had known how bad it was going to be, she would have taken the day off, but she had just started her shift and couldn't leave.

Then we tried to get a private-duty nurse for Ray that night; none was available. So Cindy, Betsy, and Cathy stayed with him, while Holly came home with me. She was thoroughly worn out, emotionally and physically. The girls kept me informed throughout the night and, while his vital signs were stable, he was hallucinating from the sedation. The next morning Gina, Holly, and I took shifts from 6:00 a.m on, and at 10:30 a.m., we were asked to leave so he could sleep.

After lunch Ray was doing better. The color was returning to his face. Dr. Thomas stopped in to check him. When he mentioned another dose of the chemo in four weeks, I thought, "God help us all." However, I knew in my heart that there could be no more of it.

On August 1 we brought Ray home. He slept most of that day and the following. We didn't even mention food around him. He couldn't eat and was only able to tolerate a little bit of fluids. His lungs were clear, but he was still coughing constantly, which caused vomiting because of the nausea. It went on and on in a vicious cycle. I sat with him and could do nothing but just be there. He couldn't hold the morphine down in liquid form any more, so tomorrow we would have to start injecting it. Betsy was going to show me how.

At that point I felt a strong need to make Ray a new tape, different from the aggressive orca tape. I meditated first, asking for guidance, and amazingly my words poured out in a great rush. On the tape, I took Ray on a journey in a blue and white airplane through the quiet sky, then farther on through the galaxy, among the stars and into the serenity of outer space. As soon as he heard the tape, he slipped quickly into the guided meditation and, when he came back, he was wearing a knowing smile.

He told me it had given him a good feeling and eased the pain, too. He had seen himself among the planets, traveling into the outer reaches of space. It made me deeply happy that I had been able to help him by creating the tape. I knew from his facial expression that my guided meditation had prompted him to also make a trip into the spiritual realms. I was on his wavelength, and he knew it. It wasn't necessary to verbalize it.

The tape was my way of letting him know that I was aware of where he was mentally and emotionally. I added a finishing touch then. I found a small, wooden model plane, painted it blue and white, and printed his initials on the fuselage. Then I hung it by a piece of thread from the ceiling over his bed. He watched it as it moved slightly to and fro, pushed by the soft breaths of breeze coming in through the open window near his bed. The other two pictures—of the plane and the sandy beach—were hanging close on the wall, and the white orca that Cindy had painted for him sat beside him on the nightstand. Fluffy, the cat, had been keeping vigil on the chair next to Ray's bed, carefully observing everything he did. Orie, my elkhound, had remained in Ray's room ever since he came home.

Ray was so quiet and peaceful. All he wanted was for me to be near him. It was late. He had just completed his new tape again and was free of pain. Since he got sick, I had begun sleeping in the adjoining room, although sometimes I laid next to him for a nap. That night I lay in our bed with him, holding his hand until he drifted off. Through contact with his hand I began to sense something extraordinary. Waves of slow expansion and contraction now emanated from him and seemed to wash over me. His vibrations swept me up and carried me slowly along a curving rise and fall, as if mighty breaths were being breathed in and out with universal widening.

Later, after Ray fell asleep, I lay very still and kept reminding myself not to move. I was afraid to fall asleep, so I would close my eyes for a few minutes to try to drift into that special time and space before sleep. I was still holding his hand, feeling the slow, widening vibrations that his body was radiating, and I joined him in that place where he was, encountering dark floating images and valleys and mountains and lights—mass chaos without meaning. The images went on and on. The experience wasn't frightening, but I didn't understand it. The amount of chaos soon became overwhelming. I felt like an intruder. Finally, near dawn, I got up and walked around, trying to clear myself. Then, I went back to the bed in the other room, so I wouldn't disturb him and I tried to sleep.

Ray slept most of the day and woke up in the evening. He was still telling me that he was not ready to give up. I told him not to worry about us; he had admitted to me that leaving us alone, without him, was a great concern of his. It was important to me that he not worry about us. I wanted to give him permission to leave, and I sensed that the time was right to verbalize it. I also told him to just do whatever he had to do, that he would be fine, that we would all be fine, too. He seemed somewhat relieved to hear that. It seemed perfectly natural for us to express these thoughts now. There was no two-way meaning or any holding back of the direct, simple truth. We had entered a place where only truth was allowed. Ray was so tired now, and I could feel him slipping slowly away from me.

On August 5, my friend Joanne, who had been with me initially when Ray was diagnosed, stopped by to visit. She and Betsy were in the kitchen when I got home from the market. Betsy took my bag of groceries.

"How come you bought coffee ice cream and root beer?" she asked with surprise. "Remember how Grandma Jessie loved this? She used to make root beer floats all summer long. We haven't had them in years."

Betsy turned to put the ice cream in the freezer, while I remained stunned because I hadn't consciously realized what I had bought. Without noticing the label, I had chosen coffee ice cream instead of vanilla. What made it doubly strange was that I had forgotten to get soda, so as I was exiting at the check-out counter, I spotted some soda nearby and grabbed what was there.

With Betsy's reminder of my mother, an image flashed quickly through my mind. I saw her dipping into her root beer float for the ice cream. The hair on my arms and back stood straight up. Joanne said softly, "My *God*, your *mother's* here. Look at my arm!" I looked over at her and saw that the hair on her arm was straight up, too, as if electricity had shot through her. Then to my amazement, Joanne proceeded to describe my mother's physical appearance accurately, even though my mother was deceased and Joanne had never met her.

Suddenly we realized that my mother, Jessie, had come back to help Ray. He had encountered her last January, nearly eight months before, during his vision in the den. During it, she had asked him about his "bout." I remembered she had told him he would be all cleared up in about a year, and she would see him later. I sensed that she was letting me know that she was here to help him. Joanne told me that for the past few days she felt that Ray had definitely made his choice.

I was soon injecting Ray with morphine every three to four hours. One day he said he was so tired of being sick, he couldn't even remember what it felt like to be well. I wept for such a long time that night that I thought there could be no more tears left.

On Friday, August 8, Ray woke up with his breathing very labored. Even though he managed to get to the bathroom, he nearly didn't make it back into bed. His pulse was rapid and thready, and he had nearly collapsed from the short trip. I called the girls early and asked them to come over. The visiting nurse had stopped by at about 8:00 a.m. to check Ray over. She ordered a hospital bed for him so he would be more comfortable.

When I got up that morning, I knew there were three things I had to do. It was so intense in my mind I couldn't rest until I got them done. First, I had to get Ray's mother over to the house to see him. Then, I had to call a priest. Lastly, I had to call the funeral parlor. I knew he would be leaving us within the next few days; of this I was certain.

I felt that I had separated into different parts and that the physical body was working now, while the rest of me was just floating along. I heard myself speaking to the funeral parlor director very calmly, like there was a stranger speaking out from inside me. It was necessary for me to know what their procedure was in the event that Ray left us in the middle of the night or near dawn. Strong inner feelings told me that this would happen, that I needed a sense of order. The funeral director was most kind; he remembered me from when my mother died. He told me that he was on twenty-four-hour call and not to worry about the financial arrangements; we could take care of things later. He was a kind man, and I appreciated his response.

I suddenly realized that maybe my emotional self wasn't just floating along; it was calm. Was it because I had accepted that Ray's sad journey was nearly over? Or was I thankful that he would soon be out of the terrible misery that he had suffered through these long, long months? Or was it the Holy Spirit, my constant companion, that was once more coming to my aid? I wasn't quite sure what was happening, but I was suspicious of the serenity and suspected that suppressed emotions were lurking at a deep inner level, marking time, like a volcano waiting to erupt.

Ray nodded to me when I asked his permission to call the priest. My childhood conditioning in Catholicism was strong. Since this trauma was so great, I was still driven to call the

priest. Birth and death, baptism and last rites were still important, and, to me, these sacraments still blessed the coming in
and the going out. It proved that I had not detached completely from the church. Even though I knew it would
probably make no difference to Ray, I needed the priest to
visit. I was sure Ray knew that I needed that.

The priest came by later. Two of my daughters were upset,
feeling that it was hypocritical of me because they knew there
was a lot that I could not accept in the church's teachings.
However, what the men of the church taught had always been
inconsequential to me. I believed in my heart that Jesus was
an advanced soul, sent from God as Master here on earth. He
had brought the Christ Consciousness to all people and the
Holy Spirit was the heralder of God's kingdom on earth. So, in
my mind, God was indeed Father, Son, and Holy Spirit, representing different parts of the whole, each being a whole unto
itself; the rituals were merely symbolic of that.

The priest asked us to join hands around Ray's bed in a
prayer gathering called Sacrament of the Sick (instead of last
rites). Two of the girls wouldn't join the gathering, so we were
divided. There were angry words afterward, then I dismissed
it. To me, that night, the theological issues just weren't important.

Later in the day, I collected Ray's mother and brought her
over. She had to be coaxed, however, because it meant facing
reality, but I was insistent and she did come.

Friday came to an end, with the evening slowly giving way
to darkness. The girls were all there. We put a cot in Ray's
room, so I could remain there with him. His hospital bed was
near the window where he wanted to be, and he could look
out. I tried to get some sleep and dozed on and off fitfully. At
4:30 a.m. Saturday morning, Ray woke me up and asked me
to sit with him.

"Put some lights on," he said. "It's so dark in here."

I switched on the soft light near the bed on the nightstand and sat quietly with him, holding his hand. We both knew what was about to happen. We found no need for words to express it. The time was for something else. We felt each other's presence acutely, our senses finely tuned to one another, connecting in a spiritual plane that was deep and ancient and binding. The silence and the place where we both were was beautiful, and communication was at a sensory level where we were no longer solitary. I was where he was, he was at peace, and I was able to truly accept what he had to do.

We had talked about sending each other a sign if we were ever parted. I didn't want to press him earlier when we had spoken of it, but now it was so vitally important to me, I asked him. He smiled just a little and said, "I'll send you a great white fleet of dolphins." I was surprised that he didn't say orcas, but he was acutely aware of what he was saying. Then he looked at me closely and said, "I want to thank you for being so kind to me."

It was his way of telling me that he was getting ready to leave. I wept spontaneously, but he comforted me and was strong. I didn't want him to leave, but I knew that he had to. I told him again that I would go with him in a minute, because I knew where he was going. I reminded him of the place I had seen in my cosmic dream. I said that I had things left here to do and that I had to stay. He nodded and said he knew that, too.

The expansive vibrations that I had been feeling from him continued: a great slowing down and widening, a huge gradual contraction, in and out with a rhythm that I had never experienced before when touching someone. It didn't frighten me, but then I had never felt anything like it before. The feelings I had been sensing from him early that morning were becoming more intense: soft and contracting vibrations, rolling in like large, softened waves of energy. It was dawning on me that this was Ray's spirit coming to the fore, drawing his "all" back into its custody through gigantic breaths, expanding slowly in and out. We sat quietly, then, holding hands; the depth of understanding between us conveyed in the sound of silence.

Something remarkable occurred at that moment and continued for several minutes. The physical room seemed to recede and become almost an illusion. I was aware of my body, but I seemed to be out of my body, intensely shifting focus at that moment into a place that up to that moment had only given me occasional fleeting glimpses of itself in dreams. I felt expansive and encompassing simultaneously. Ray was with me in that familiar place. The world had receded, and we were drawn into a deep plane of serenity; alone together, but safe.

We found ourselves communicating at a spiritual level, deeply, and the experience was truly astounding. It didn't last very long, but we had touched at the level of an extraordinary awareness. In those few brief minutes I understood fully that whatever had happened or whatever would happen from here on regarding the physical was not really important. We had been given the privilege of taking part in a communion of our souls at that very moment. It was a precious gift from above; it was true and it was real. I had sensed correctly from the beginning: Ray had chosen this route, not to end his physical body but to heal all the hurt from his early life that he had never been given the tools to fix. He had finally learned to be free and communicated with me totally, at last. We were of one heart on that plane of serenity, and his lifelong communication problem was now over.

For the first time in thirty-three years I knew the deepest recesses of his heart. I saw the rooms of his broken inner house swept clean and the windows of his soul finally open. Whatever problems or traumas we had experienced across our earth years together didn't matter any more; they had been washed away. Most of them had been physical and fleeting, a minor part of a journey that we had chosen together. The joyous times were there for me to remember and hold closely in my heart. The moment was *now*, the only precious moment of real import. We had shared the good and the bad throughout our lifetime, but never a serious thought of breaking our bond. Our physical adventure together was wide and varying. I believed that we had experienced more in this life than most do in many. But that was what life here was all about; we had chosen a journey, and now Ray was at his terminus, ready to disembark. He had chosen to end the dance; he had completed his part, but I knew that I would have to continue on.

His spirit was trying to gain freedom from its physical trap, which was only the vehicle he had used for this fleeting earth life. We were truly players on a great stage, and the exit was near for him. I felt that he had taken on so much in this lifetime, for reasons known only to his soul. It had taken all of his spiritual energy to survive the really great battle he had come here to do. Our quiet and deep communion that night had answered a lot of questions concerning our relationship over the years. His soul had been intensely focused on this life's mission, which had required great spiritual energy. How much could he work on in one lifetime? How many other things had he been able to focus on? Whatever he had come to do this time, he had done it.

During those brief racing moments, I was aware of the strong spiritual force within him and I touched his soul, one which was free, healed, and now ready to graduate from the karmic school which is the earth. I knew at that moment how strongly tied we really had been. My only regret was what a life-dance we could have done together if his spirit had not been so totally dominated by his personal battle.

But then again I knew it had to be. Whatever part I had chosen to help him in playing out his role, I had fulfilled it. We didn't talk about death because at that moment we understood what had to happen. It was inevitable, and it was all right. We knew we would be together again, cast in new roles, but still the same players in a new lifetime, perhaps not very far into the future. Ray's new spiritual breakthrough would carry him forth now.

Overwhelming insight had come to my mind during those precious few minutes. I had loved Ray and still loved him on a level that could not be expressed in words. The true journey that we had traveled together was the main focus, even though we had not known it consciously. I was exquisitely aware of it now and knew that he knew it, too. We continued to sit in silence, me never wanting the moment to end, and he now completely cognizant of all his conscious encounters with spirit.

The sun came up without us realizing it, spreading a soft golden glow over the room. Ray asked me to open the blinds and let the sun in. Then he told me to go back and lie down, that I would need my sleep. Unbelievably, I did sleep for a few hours.

As the day progressed, Cindy told us of the increasing silent activity going on around us. She expressed it as expansiveness. She described the many small white lights she saw moving about her father, and the shadowy guide-like shapes present in the room. Probably the expansiveness that she spoke of was what I had been feeling during the past two days.

Toward the afternoon, Ray lost ground rapidly. He was too weak to even talk, so I called Dr. Thomas about 4:00 p.m. I told him again that Ray could not eat and that he could only hold liquids down. Dr. Thomas advised me that he could take Ray back into the hospital and get nourishment into him through an I.V.—but that would only prolong the inevitable for about three or four days. By law, he had to inform me of what he was able to do medically. Dr. Thomas said that, personally, he would do what we were doing, that Betsy could administer more morphine if Ray asked for it. Ray had expressed his need to be with me at home, and this wish would be honored.

I felt I should tell Ray what the doctor had said. I told him, but he didn't answer me. I knew he had heard me, yet I repeated it again. The second time he ignored it, too; then I didn't say any more. I knew in my heart that Ray would leave us early the next morning. He was tired and finished here, and I agreed with his choice. I was then in a consciousness where I knew what he wanted. I had experienced something wondrous and rare, especially between two people for whom communication had always been so hard in coming.

CHAPTER ELEVEN

CONSCIOUS ENCOUNTERS WITH SPIRIT

(August)

It was evening now, Saturday, August 9, and Ray was slowly beginning to disconnect from the earth. We all knew what was transpiring and flowed with him, as if the tide were coming in to take him back out, and he was merging with it. There was no confusion among us, only a melding with him, following his lead, just being there with him.

The healer, Mary, had told me that it was important to assure him that he was doing everything right and that all was going well and was as it should be. The reassurance helped him; he showed no fear or apprehension. He had been refusing the morphine since early afternoon and told me he didn't need it. He wouldn't sleep and managed to keep his eyes wide open. Betsy's friend Becky, who is an R.N., was with us. She had brought drops for his eyes. We were concerned because he would not blink, and the drops were needed to keep his eyes moist. If I spoke to him, he would usually focus back to the room, but he was definitely present elsewhere. It was such an intense concentration; his lips moved, silently mouthing words, and we knew surely that he was speaking with someone. His focus was slowly starting to shift out of the room into some other time and place. It was such a personal and profound happening for him that I couldn't bring myself to interrupt. I only asked him one question:

"Is Christina there to help you?"

It was extremely difficult for him to alter his focal point, but he shifted his eyes to mine and answered, "Yes." At that moment, the knowledge that he would leave us at 3:00 a.m. passed into my mind. Now I understood why I had been so intensely guided to call the funeral home. He would cross over in the early hours of the morning on August 10.

We sat with him all evening and tried to make him comfortable. He was able to sip water in drops through a straw which Holly held for him. The spiritual activity increased around him. Cindy and I saw many guide shapes, outlined softly against the wall, filling the space in the room. As the twilight darkened into night, he remained conscious, eyes wide open, but his focus was not there in the room. It was as though he were being absorbed into another place, but the transference was not happening all at once. A slow disconnecting from the physical was occurring.

"Dad doesn't want us all here watching him. I just know it," Holly whispered to me.

I asked Ray about that; he nodded his head, yes. We were wondering if he would permit us all to be with him because he was such a private person. I knew I would stay, but perhaps he didn't want everyone there. The girls went out of the room for awhile and I remained, holding his hand. In a little while, two of my daughters came back in; they hadn't been able to stay away. Then the other two slipped back in, also. It was then that Ray decided to permit us all to be with him through the long hushed hours of his last night with us.

We drifted slowly in and out of the gentle, quiet minutes as the night deepened now, past midnight, past 1:00 a.m., when a breathless quiet filled the room. Since early afternoon he had only been able to whisper, but suddenly and with great vocal force he said to me loudly, "Let go of my hand!"

It stunned me for a moment, but I knew immediately why he was saying this to me. I quickly let go. I sincerely thought I had fully accepted that he was leaving and that I would not try to hold him here, but it was hard being ordered by him to let go. I was only human. I wasn't hanging on consciously. I was tuned in deeply to him. Although I was quite calm at that moment, we were entwined at an inner level which I hadn't recognized and some part of my energy was anchoring him.

Cindy said his vibrations were starting to change more rapidly; he was tuning in to a different wavelength, so to speak, and I sensed then that my earth energies were blocking and interfering with his new vibrations. Then I was afraid to touch him, so I just sat near him in silence.

Cindy turned on the stereo and played the soft ethereal music of Kitaro's *Silk Road*, which filled the room with a spiritual lightness. I was sitting by the side of the bed, very close to him, but not touching him. He was so intense, his lips still mouthing words which we could not understand. I glanced at the clock. It was 2:15 a.m. At that second, I was compelled to take myself out of the room. My conscious mind did not understand because I didn't want to leave, but I had no choice or control. Something powerful had overruled my ego. A moment later, I found myself standing in the bathroom, sobbing. What was happening? Why was I doing this when he was so close to leaving? I didn't understand, and it was frightening for me to have lost mastery of my ego.

While I was standing in the bathroom those few minutes, not knowing why I was there, Cindy later told me what had transpired. Ray had been motionless for some time, but then he suddenly squeezed Betsy's and Cindy's hands forcefully. As he did this, Betsy felt a shock wave like electricity move up her arm with great intensity; Cindy felt an abrupt change of vibration in his hand, and a great surge of energy and lightness was transferred into her. Then Cindy saw a swirling vortex emanating from his head, reaching to the ceiling above. She said it was like seeing a whirling motion in clear water; with this, he turned his palms upward. He was still deeply concentrating, trancelike.

Suddenly Cindy called to me, "Mom. They're here for him."

The spell was broken. I rushed back into the room and sat down on the chair I had left a few minutes before. As I sat down, I was nearly lifted physically from the chair. The room had somehow changed. A soft radiant glow was present. The energy was electrifying and overwhelming. I sensed an omnipotent force around us but I could only see immense vague outlines.

The energy in the room was so powerful that I felt that the Holy Spirit had entered to take him. My heart started to beat rapidly; I was terribly afraid. A thought shot through my mind at that moment of the Biblical accounts of actual encounters with the Holy Spirit. I knew what "sorely afraid" meant. I wish I could convey in words the force and power of the Holy Spirit that we experienced that night. Yet, I realized the fear was only in my body because of my ego. I was suddenly extremely aware of the separation of spirit and ego in myself.

The guide activity increased rapidly with the energy and with the phenomenon of the Holy Spirit. It was all so frightening, yet so spiritually beautiful that it took my breath away. Then a great calm and peace enveloped me, gentling my heart, taking the fear, and lifting me into incredible lightness. Cindy saw all manner of forms and outlines and swirling cone-shapes in the electrifying radiance of the room.

My awareness came back to the physical. I glanced at the clock on the nightstand; it was approaching 3:00 a.m. The energy was still in the room, but its intensity was gone. Ray's breathing became more shallow, and at about 3:07 a.m. I sensed a definite shift, as did Betsy. She told us that he was leaving.

We all huddled closer, holding him as best we could. My last words to him were to look for the light and that I loved him. The girls each told him good-by and how much they loved him and that we would see him again. He took three deep breaths, turned to Betsy sitting next to him, closed his eyes, and finally slipped through "God's other door." He did it with such dignity, so fearlessly, we could not realize for the moment that he was gone. We knew that he had crossed safely and without fear. His great lion heart simply stopped along with his breathing. Betsy could not believe that he had closed his eyes on his own and said to him softly, "You did it right, Dad."

She later told us that that usually didn't happen after the eyes had been opened for nearly twelve hours. He had done everything so peacefully that we just sat for a long moment, stunned, unable to comprehend that we had just witnessed a radiant passage.

Then our humanness rushed back in. We realized what had happened. Yes, we had been privileged to participate in that powerful spiritual wonderment, but we knew then that we had lost him. He was gone physically from us forever, and the finality, which right then we could not perceive fully, began to creep in. The long intense months of the sickness gave way to the peaceful crossing over. It burst into our consciousness like a clap of thunder. His journey had ended; here was his terminus; he had been released, but we had to continue on without him. I was completely drained. The spiritual energy that had visited the room was like a nuclear power plant compared to our tiny nightlights. The experience had depleted us; no one could move.

The room was hushed and very still. The world had stopped for us. We quietly said our tearful final good-bys to him. We still could not fully acknowledge what had just occurred. It was intensely private for each of us, never to be accurately shared. Cindy offered the thought that she believed his soul had left earlier than the death of his physical body. She felt that his soul crossed over when the intensity of the radiant energy was at a peak. We agreed with her and realized that we had all had a magnificent and glorious final conscious encounter together.

It was nearly 4:00 a.m. when we left the room to go downstairs to sit in the den. Holly stayed a few minutes longer with her father, then joined us. Someone had called the funeral parlor and, because none of us could sit still too long, some of us wandered outside to wait for them to arrive. In the quiet stillness before dawn, we sat on the front steps. I felt completely detached, as if my physical body were functioning alone without any direction.

They took Ray's body away at 5:00 a.m. We lingered in the den a while longer in detached numbness. Each of us was completely lost in our own thoughts in the quiet room when Betsy's daughter, eight-year-old Sarah wandered downstairs, crying. She had been looking for her Pop-Pop and couldn't find him. She said his bed was empty and that she knew he had died. Sarah never woke up in the middle of the night. She had kissed and hugged him last evening before she went to bed. I was so thankful that she hadn't awakened earlier.

We roamed about the house aimlessly, not knowing what to do. No one could sleep, so we went up to one of the other bedrooms and sat on the bed together. Gina brought a decanter of brandy with her. None of us were drinkers, but we thought this perhaps would help us attach back to the physical. We talked softly until the bright morning sun invaded our inner sanctum. Then we got up to face the long dreadful day that lay ahead.

The first week after Ray died was crowded with strange events. We each at various times felt pockets of heat in the kitchen, which had been more like a family room where we often gathered together. Twice I checked the thermostat to see if the heat had been turned on. Even though it was summer, the temperature was markedly different in the kitchen than in the rest of the house. I kept asking if someone had turned the heat on. Then I remembered the etheric body and how sometimes it takes the personality longer to leave. Was Ray being drawn to the family gathering room?

We felt his presence so strongly when we were all together. It was like turning around, expecting to see someone behind you or catching a glimpse of a presence just outside your peripheral vision, but there is no one there. Cindy, our visual, saw him a number of times. She said he was happy and well; we all knew that he was experimenting with his new-found freedom. I felt he was concerned about us and told him that we would be okay, that he didn't have to worry. Then I sensed that he was more at peace.

We decided on cremation for Ray's body. He had been a pilot and loved the sky. He adored soaring over the earth, so we could not put him under the earth. In the meantime, I was completely devastated. I didn't know how I would get through the memorial service we had planned for the following week.

We had asked Lou to conduct the service, and he was pleased that we had done so. It was going to be difficult for us, but we wished to plan it the way Ray would have wanted. Lou told us that a funeral service is a necessary and important ritual. It is more than just tradition, and has a much deeper meaning. The dead must be sealed off from the earth so that they can journey onward, without being held here. The bond to the material world has to be broken; the emotional ties must be severed by the departed; friends and family have to clear themselves of anything that has not been resolved with the one who is now in spirit. The dead have to leave, unencumbered, to freely continue on their path. In this way, friends and family are allowed to open their hearts and heal what has been left undone.

Lou said that this is part of the ancient meaning behind funeral rites. We also had to remember that it was harder for those of us left behind; the departed ones were now reborn back into spirit, so it was a happy time for them. In our hearts we completely agreed, but it was so hard being human and having to be without Ray.

We decided to hold the memorial service in the little white clapboard church on the next block, right here in our small town. Each of us wanted to write our own eulogy, and together we would choose the music. Lou would invite anyone to join us who wished to express personal thoughts. It was traumatic for us when we stopped for a minute to realize just what we were doing, but organizing and planning the memorial service occupied our time, giving us something to do.

One week later the girls and I walked into the church and were stunned to see it filled to capacity. I guess we hadn't thought about who would come. We all had many friends; some people were even standing in the back of the overflowing church. The love present that day was overwhelming. I hoped that somehow we would get through it without breaking down. I unconsciously looked around for Ray because I felt his presence so strongly.

As I sat down in the first bench, my eyes were drawn upward to an enormous red silk tapestry, about twenty feet square, hanging on the wall behind the pulpit. At first I saw many outlines and shapes etched against the red silk. As I continued to stare, the shapes seemed to merge into one form. It was a gigantic outline of a man sitting on a large chair. The face and top of the body were in profile, a silhouette similar to that of an Egyptian pharaoh or a bishop with a conelike hat or crown on his head. He was seated on his throne, and he was huge. I was stunned for the moment and kept staring at the tapestry. The profile grew more distinct and did not waver. It remained steadfast throughout the entire ceremony and did not fade.

Cindy tearfully read her eulogy to her father. Holly attempted hers, but she was unable to go on. Lou completed Holly's for her, then read mine, Betsy's, and Gina's. I knew that Ray was there, listening to our farewells and communicating inwardly with all his friends. We were pleased that some also voiced their remembrances of Ray. I fully realized then what a funeral rite should be and what it was meant to accomplish.

When the service was finally over, Annmarie hugged me. Without knowing what I had seen, she told me she saw Ray, looking like Zeus sitting on his throne. Four other friends described similar sights that they had seen in the church. I knew that what I saw on the red fabric was real. Cindy, too, had seen outlines and shapes on the tapestry and felt that they were spirit guides who had come to help, manifesting themselves there.

After the service, everyone came back to the house in the old tradition. My neighbors and friends had been so kind; the table was laden with food. I could not allow myself to think about the days, weeks, and months ahead. I just wasn't ready to deal with the thought of going on without Ray.

The next week continued to bring unusual paranormal incidents with Ray sending us help and comfort. Holly had a dream about him set in an ancient time. She and he were mates in the dream, and this was very specific—*mates*. She didn't know if she had been the male or the female, and it really didn't make any difference, she said. They were sitting on a rock somewhere, and he was telling her something or trying to explain something to her about the meaning of existence. They loved each other very much. It had given Holly comfort seeing him again in this dream. I remembered Edgar Cayce's statement that memory reveals itself some time after death, not only the immediate past life but all memory is recalled for introspection by the newly departed. Perhaps Ray had been recalling a former life with Holly, and she tuned in to it.

Gina also had a dream in which she was sitting with Ray in her room. They were both looking through the connecting door to another room, where Ray's body was lying on the bed. She was frightened. Ray assured her that he was all right, that it was just his physical body. Then in her room she saw his face and part of his body while they were sitting together. He had a cut on his face that he had gotten while shaving. He told her he had to go take care of it. Perhaps he had chosen to present himself to her in a more familiar way, even down to the shaving cut, so as not to frighten her. I remembered when Gina was small, how she loved to watch her father shave. Gina was happy that she had seen him and that he told her that he was happy. She realized that he was telling her that only his body was dead, but his soul had continued on.

Ray's final farewell to me turned out to be both unsettling and beautiful. The night after the memorial service I went to visit Cindy. My car was parked on the side street next to the house, facing the eastern horizon. I was worn down, drained of energy, and for the first time too tired to be anything but calm. My mind was not cranking and whirling; no thoughts were racing through my head. I opened the car door, got in, and sat down behind the steering wheel. As I put the key into the ignition, however, I simultaneously looked up through the windshield and the sight took my breath away. I couldn't understand what I was seeing. The moon was down so low, appeared so huge and close that it was covering and almost completely obliterating the horizon. The entire area in front of me was filled with the moon's pale yellow light.

What I was seeing directly in front of me made no sense. I sat frozen, confused, and unable to comprehend. It was like a scene from a science fiction movie, and I knew it couldn't be real. Yet, there it was before my eyes. I could see the moon's canals and markings in great detail and thought it had to be the end of the world! That was the only logic I could apply. My next thought was that the moon had spun off course and was about to collide with the earth. I wondered if the earth would be knocked out of orbit. I became terribly disoriented. The thought crossed my mind that maybe I was asleep and dreaming.

I was desperately trying to apply sanity to a completely insane event. I had to warn everyone, and I didn't know if there was time to do it. But I felt I had to try. I consciously forced myself to turn away, as I felt for the door handle to get out of the car. But when I looked again a split second later, everything was back to normal. The full, light golden moon was riding high in the sky where it belonged. Now I just sat, stuck to the seat, terribly shaken, thinking that I had lost my mind for sure. Then I heard Ray. I heard him distinctly, just as if he were sitting next to me. He said, "You can't imagine what it's like!"

Then I knew with absolute certainty how free he really was and that his journey here on this plane was over. What a send-off! Still dazed, I ran into the house to tell the girls. I assumed it had to be some kind of psychic occurrence; I was curious to know what had happened. I felt that somehow I had been seeing what Ray was seeing.

Holly and Cindy each had beautiful farewell experiences with clouds and rays of sunshine. They felt that Ray was trying to show them just how happy he was.

A few weeks later I called Annmarie and asked her to do a reading for me. I wanted more precise answers from another source to the many questions I had about Ray's passing. I was especially eager to know why I seemed to have no control when I left the room just before Ray was ready to cross. But there was more. I also wanted to know what exactly it was that Cindy saw when his soul departed, what Ray was trying to present to us in the church, and the meaning of my strange observation of the moon. I was anxious, now that Ray had left us, to see if Josef could give us any more information about Ray's mission in this lifetime. So I asked him what part karma had played in Ray's illness. He answered with the following:

> "First, I would like to say that I do not hold to the popular idea of karma. I do not hold that you must pay with an eye for an eye, meaning the exact same retribution for past debts. The soul does require certain lessons to encourage its journey. Human beings are a stubborn lot, and they will remain complacent until life sort of ejects them into growth.
>
> "Take someone who has never had trial or tribulation; someone who is undeveloped. So, a lot of things in Raymond's life happened around him. They happened to others, and he was directly affected, but it was not something that happened within his consciousness. So, he lived his life often as an observer and had reactions to what he observed.
>
> "Many of those reactions emotionally were repressed. Well, in the final time of his life, he took on something deeply personal, something internal, something wholly his, and moved a great deal. In doing so, he did not choose to get cancer . . . but he contracted for a long-term illness that would lead to his crossing. He did that because he needed time before he crossed."

Josef said that if Ray had crossed abruptly, several things would have occurred. He would not have reached the level he was on now, and he would have been angry. Josef also said that I would not have survived it, and our daughters would have suffered even more. Ray had done this in a way that enabled him to see everyone through while maintaining his own spiritual integrity. And, Josef continued, he took the personality to the next level, actually doing an *intensive* for spiritual growth. That word seemed to say it all.

The important thing, Josef suggested, was not to dwell on

that seven-and-a-half-month span of time in which Ray had been ill, not to think of it as being a time of development or a hardship. He advised me to just let the period go and allow myself to experience the flow of it.

I asked Josef if he could tell me why Ray chose to do an "intensive," and he answered:

> "It took this intensive to break the defenses he had built around himself. The defenses were there so that he could get through the life; then he broke them down in order to end the life. But if he had broken them down and not crossed over, you still would not have gotten what you had bargained for, because he would have spent many years being angry. Your marriage may not have survived it, the struggle he would have had to go through; so he broke it down through illness. He let his body take it, as I told you before; the body took it and the suffering was less."

I questioned Josef on why Ray had needed such tremendous defenses in life. He told me that Raymond had not been loved as a child. That created a great deal of anger, and he'd had a rage within him that was murderous in his mind. He had to suppress that and was afraid of what he would do if he ever tapped into it. Josef went on to say that it was not only rage from Ray's childhood, but that past lives were also involved. He said that Ray had several choices, that he chose the best one, and—though it was hard to understand—the least painful way of doing it.

> "He took you all on a very exciting journey. So, the other way, the way you would have preferred, would have been hard and long and not as fulfilling, and he still might not have reached his spiritual

fulfillment by dealing with the emotional. This way he dealt with all levels at once in a short period of time, and the suffering was condensed, as opposed to drawn out over time."

Then I asked why I had accompanied him in his terrible journey. Josef told me that we had been together many times, and I had contracted with Ray in this lifetime so that we could support each other as we progressed to the next level of our spiritual development. Ray had supported me while I sought to heal my past through therapy, but he had chosen to remain behind. Josef continued, saying that I had supported Ray during those seven months and that Ray was grateful for my helping him to cross so easily.

Josef then related a message to us from Ray. Ray said that his transition had been quite easy. He wanted his girls to know that, even though he was going to be involved in many new endeavors, a part of him would always live inside of them and he would always surround them with his love. He said that if they should ever wish to communicate with him, they could do so; all they had to do was call to him aloud, and he would answer them in some way—through a dream, in their thoughts, or whatever they would be open to.

Continuing the reading, Josef said that Ray wanted me to know that he was available to me, too, but he felt that I, for a change, was blocking communications with *him*. He said there was nothing to be afraid of and that he only wished to console me. I explained to Josef that I was concerned that I would hold him here if I tried to reach out to him too often. I had felt him around so frequently that I was worried about this and wanted him to be free. Josef explained that what I had been feeling was the etheric body—the personality—that was around, adding that the warm spots in the kitchen we had experienced was Ray's etheric body. He said that Ray's soul had gone immediately.

I mentioned the fact that I had not asked to see Ray in my dreams because of the same reason. Josef told me that, despite my conscious concerns, I had made it clear that I didn't want to be stimulated then and that this was my subconscious way of protecting myself. Ray had transcended the personality and, therefore, no longer possessed fear. So he wanted to greet me right away, whereas I, still being on the earth plane, needed to be a little more cautious.

I told Josef that I was puzzled when Ray told me to let go of his hand. I had moved away without wanting to, and Cindy had moved in next to him. Josef answered that it wasn't so much that Cindy needed to move in; it was more that I had to move away to create a space for him to go, that our energies were so entwined that he couldn't get free from his body. He had been rocking and rocking, and he hadn't been able to get out. By my leaving, he was able to lift.

I asked him if my mother had come to help Ray cross over and Josef affirmed it. Then I asked about Christina. Josef said that "It was just a part of her" and that she was also a guide to Holly. I understood that to mean that Christina, the spiritual guide presented to Ray, was only a small part of the entity's essence. Another part of her was a guide to Holly. I wondered if she had also been part of Ray's essence.

I asked Josef what Ray would be doing now that he was on another plane. He told me that he was going to be "helping to hold the vibration steady, helping individuals, and acting not so much as a guide, but as a source of strength for them to tap into." He was also going to be doing a lot of evaluating of his previous lifetimes. I recalled again that the Cayce readings suggest that there is a period of time after the transition which we spend doing just that, seeing whether we can finish up on the other side or whether we have to return to another life on earth. Josef confirmed for me that Holly's dream about her father, in which they were together in ancient times, was indeed a past-life memory.

I wanted to get an accurate explanation of my psychic experience with the moon, so I asked Josef to explain what happened. What he said made me feel a lot more comfortable about the event.

> "Your aura, as you would call it, opened up and allowed you to see where Raymond was going. But you didn't see it through his eyes; it was just an opening in space."

"What did I experience in the church?" I asked. Josef immediately told me that Raymond thought he would be "king of the castle." Josef had a sense of humor, but he was also right on target. We had all kidded Ray about that because of his living with five women. The girls had even made him a crown after that margarine commercial came out years ago.

Josef told me that Ray didn't want me to continue thinking of him now in the depleted bodily state that he was in when he left us. He wanted to appear to us in his true form, so we would see him as he really is. The others who were present at the memorial service weren't able to see what I had seen on the tapestry, but many perceived the feeling that Ray was conveying—that something much larger was going on. Ray's ravaged physical image had been deeply etched into our minds. It was horrendous for us to remember him that way, so this message in particular helped us immensely.

I realized that Ray's illness and passing had helped me raise my level of spiritual awareness, but I didn't know what to do with it or how to pass it on to others. I wished that I could make use of all the inner knowledge I had acquired and now felt it was my responsibility to do so. I asked Josef what I could do about it. He said:

> "Well, you can do it in several ways. You can write a series of articles and send them to various

magazines. In this way you would be helping people. Or you could write a book. Another idea, which you're not yet ready for but some day you might consider, is counseling in a cancer ward or, if not cancer, then some other form of helping ill people motivate themselves toward health."

I related the magnificent cosmic dream that I had had seven months before when Ray first got ill and asked Josef why I ever chose to leave that beautiful realm. He gave me some insightful answers that helped me understand more about reincarnation and karma.

"You came to work through a portion of your own consciousness. It's interrelated and intertwined with the girls and their lives and what you all came to do together, and what you and Raymond came to do. There was a lot of interconnections between you and Betsy. I try to call them by *your* names; but you have had many, many lifetimes where you held a consciousness of a certain way, being *the* way, and in this lifetime you broke that. This was part of it. Another reason was to find strength in vulnerability, which is something that you had quite a lot of difficulty with in many lifetimes."

Josef had one final message for me, saying that in this life I had also made some deep connections with those around me. Those connections were actually what I had come to accomplish, especially my association with Ray. Therefore, he said, I had achieved a great deal in this life.

It was wonderful to have so many of our experiences confirmed and explained. I felt that Ray was happy and free.

Cindy saw Annmarie some time later, mainly to ask about what she had seen when her father left. Josef told her that she had indeed been privileged to watch her father's soul leave in the vortex of energy. Cindy felt that that was true and thanked her father for such a precious parting gift. It had allayed considerably her own fear of death.

A short time later Cindy and Cathy were up in the mountains lying on the ground and looking up at the brilliant starlit night. Cindy said aloud, "Okay, Dad. If you can hear me, let's see a shooting star."

With that, a bright radiant star shot from one end of the sky across the horizon. She said it took their breath away. Cathy, who had also been close to Ray, then said the same thing to confirm what had just happened. She, too, received a beautiful shooting star. Perhaps only the two of them saw this and maybe it had been an illusion, but it had been a real message to them from Ray. Whatever and however it happened, it was magnificent.

We all share the feeling that Ray is relieved to be freed from the physical and is joyous where he is. We wish we could understand the full content of his choice, but we know that, as each entity must face self, this is his journey. We each have our own. We know that what his soul has chosen is the right choice for him in the grand scheme. This helps us spiritually to accept his crossing, although our humanness is still very angry, hurt, and desolate, somewhat detached from the reality here and still sometimes feeling that we have only just awakened from a bad dream.

CHAPTER TWELVE

THE OTHER SIDE OF DAWN

(The Months After)

The months immediately following Ray's death were the most difficult. Two weeks after Ray died, Holly's husband left her and their two little girls. We supported her and cried with her. It was monstrous that she should have to face such a trauma so soon after her father's death. She was adamant then about finishing her college degree and got herself back into school. Her goal was set, and we were all committed to supporting her in any way that we could.

We tried to recoup our strength during the early fall, but Cindy's birthday on November 16, Thanksgiving, and finally Ray's birthday on the 30th were still ahead of us. On Cindy's birthday we all experienced a painful void without Ray. But we leaned on each other, crying spontaneously, remembering other past birthdays. We constantly shared our memories of Ray and continued to grieve together openly. Whatever anyone felt like expressing—be it anger, love, memories, or desolation—it was permitted. Then, we would all cry together and release more grief. We discussed going out to eat on Thanksgiving. But no one was really happy with that idea, and the plan fell by the wayside. We all decided we wanted to be at home for Thanksgiving. When the day arrived, the girls,

Grandma Eva, and friends came together at my house to help us get through the day. We had a lot of sad moments, especially when Cindy took over the job of carving the turkey, but we made it through.

I thought about Ray's birthday approaching, and I felt I wanted to get away. We had been supporting Holly, had bravely faced Cindy's birthday and a dismal Thanksgiving, and thought maybe a change of scene would help. That weekend, Cindy, Cathy, Holly, and I decided to go to Virginia Beach and to the islands of Chincoteague and Assateague on Virginia's eastern shore. Ray and I had always loved the area and had been there many times before by ourselves.

We had especially loved the island of Assateague, with its wild marshy woods and free-roaming ponies. Although we had often visited the A.R.E., the girls and I didn't go there this time. We needed to be outside, roaming the beaches and visiting the little shops, trying hard to move out of our consuming grief. I had tried to reach Mr. Irion, who had been so kind and helpful to me with his correspondence, but I was disappointed to learn that he wasn't available when I was there.

While we were in Chincoteague, I was anxious to visit the different places that were familiar to me, especially the small shops and the wildlife museum. We also hoped to see again some of the wild ponies on the island of Assateague.

As I walked into one particular shop to browse, memories flooded my mind of the many times Ray and I had visited here. Suddenly my eyes were drawn to a display counter, where a large magnificent sculpture took my breath away. Two beautiful white dolphins, caught in a curving thrust as if jumping from the ocean's water, were mounted on a lovely piece of highly polished driftwood. The dolphins seemed to draw me over for a closer inspection. Ray's little smile entered through my mind's eye. I remembered his face when he told me he would send me white dolphins. It was so gorgeous and quite expensive, but I bought it anyway. It was November 30, Ray's birthday, and I heard him say again that he would send me white dolphins.

We were dreading the first Christmas, but Betsy's children Luke and Sarah, and Holly's Rachael and Lindsay needed to have their Christmas. Thankfully they kept us going. Ray had gotten deeply involved with the "Shop at Home" programs on TV while he was sick, and he had ordered some inexpensive wristwatches which arrived before he died. He asked me to put them away for the girls for Christmas. I did, and nearly forgot them. I took them out, wrapped them, and hesitantly gave them to the girls. It was so sad; we all fell apart together and had a long hard cry.

Amazingly, throughout the ordeal of Ray's illness and death, Ray's mother, Eva, had never been able to shed a tear. We hugged her into our circle that Christmas, but she was still unable to cry with us. My thoughts turned to Ray and his longtime inability to communicate his emotions. It was again emphasized to me how he had never, as a child, witnessed any kind of emotional expression except anger and fighting.

There would be no more holidays until Easter, so I plodded ahead, living my days one by one. That winter I had a difficult time getting outside and back into the flow of life. As long as I could be with my family, I was fine. But whenever I ventured out, even to the store, I felt solitary and desperately separated from the rest of the world. Fortunately, between the life insurance benefits and Betsy's sharing of the household expenses, I was able to stay home for nearly a year after Ray died. During that time I buried myself in caring for the house and my grandchildren. It was a much-needed healing time, which helped me move my fragmented self toward wholeness. Betsy was working full-time, and I was there for Sarah and Luke after school. I really didn't want to face the world yet. I just tried to put my own inner house in order.

Looking back, I feel as though I just drifted that year. There had been so many emotional and spiritual challenges that I think I was actually suffering from extreme exhaustion. It was a time for rest and recouperation, both mentally and physically, and a time for me to recapture my own power.

During that healing time, I went over and over those intense seven months in my mind. I focused on whether anything could have prevented Ray's illness and if there was anything more that could have been done for him. I came to the conclusion that medical science had done everything possible; I, too, had done everything humanly possible for him. I thought about all the events in the past, before he was sick; what I could have done for him and was so sorry that I hadn't. Just little things, like being more interested in his work and giving him more of my attention. Then I would repeatedly think about his physical suffering and focus on it, remembering the way he looked.

I recall clearly the worst time of all for me, after the first Platinol treatment. It was the darkest moment of my life when I could do nothing but exist. I had roamed the park with my dog that night, asking God to take Ray then because I couldn't endure any more and couldn't understand why he had to suffer so. It took us a long, long time to get past the physical havoc that the cancer had wreaked.

Then, after a few months, I felt the anger starting to surface. Why didn't he think about me when he made his decision to leave? I was furious that he had left me. Even though it caused me great guilt, I had no choice but to acknowledge those feelings.

I was aware, however, that it was the emotional me experiencing these intense feelings. Here again, as through Ray's entire illness, was the separation between my spirit and my emotions. I realized that emotion is from the ego; after all, I was human. My inner self never forgot the real truth of our journey and, toward the end, it had even risen up and soothed me when I needed it most. I was aware that my emotional self needed healing and alignment with my inner self. There were higher powers that would stand by me. I knew that Ray was all right. I never doubted the truth of what had happened. But I didn't know any other way to grieve, so I let the feelings come through as they manifested. I knew that the Holy Spirit understood I was human and would be there to help me. I spoke inwardly with Jesus often during that time.

I had the need to go over and over it, flowing with my feelings, until I was so immersed in my grief that it started to subside. I acknowledged that it was normal for a trauma such as losing a loved one to cause depression and despair. Then slowly, I came alive again. The depression lessened. I wanted to see what was going on in the world since I had withdrawn from it over a year before. At times, my joining into the life stream again made me feel like a traitor. How could I go out and touch the world and forget about Ray? That was another hurdle to conquer. My emotional equilibrium had been tipped, and for a long time I walked around in a daze.

The slow process of coming back and balancing myself eventually began of its own accord. I guess it started happening from feelings inside, then my psyche just kept moving forward step by step. I realized that life does indeed go on, and what I had experienced with Ray was a part of it.

Then I brought to mind all the extraordinary paranormal encounters that we had had and tried to understand what I could of them. I'm still not absolutely sure why I was given that first prophetic serpent dream at that specific time. I couldn't decipher it consciously at that time. The only rationale I can use now to relate to that dream was that it had been given to me on an inner level in order to prepare my subconscious for what was about to happen. Then my subconscious mind seeped information into my consciousness to aid me along the way. I believe that dream came to me from the Holy Spirit, the messenger of the Christ Consciousness.

The serpent dream was so powerful and startling in its symbology that I could come to no other conclusion.

There was no doubt in my mind from the beginning that my glorious cosmic dream, my amazing grace, had been given to me by the Christ Consciousness. I have always had a strong belief in the Christ Consciousness, and I've tried to integrate Jesus' expression of it into my way of thinking and functioning. Even in the most desperate times of Ray's illness, I held to my beliefs and used that foundation to get my emotional self through. I believe now, as I did then, that each soul makes its own decisions. I had prayed a lot to God just to help me see Ray through. But the thought crossed my mind, Why was I so privileged to receive God's grace from above? And then I thought, Why not? Isn't that our ultimate goal? To touch that Christ Consciousness in ourselves so it will touch us back? You don't have to hold membership in any church or religion to reach out for that glorious Consciousness. It is infinitely abundant; it is there for all of us. So open your heart and ask to receive His light and love. I believe that we make daily choices, either to try our best to follow the Light or merrily go about seeking our own gratifications. As each individual is meeting himself or herself, we will all reap that which we have sown.

Speak to that part of yourself which is your "kingdom within." Your spirit resides in that "kingdom within" and is the gateway to opening to your Christ Consciousness. This is the best way when the circumstances of life, or death, bring you to your own "dark night of the soul."

Spirit has extraordinary power to manifest earthly phenomena. I believe that Ray's extraordinary out-of-body experience, his visit with my mother, his trips into his own body, and his dreams all came from his own spirit or higher self, manifesting help for him in many different ways. His inner visualization journeys and his meetings with Christina were truly astonishing. I believe all these were accomplished by focusing, through meditation, into his own realm of the spirit. The fruits of Ray's many encounters were abundant and positive. That is the real test of whether or not these encounters were holy and from the Light. I would emphasize again that meditation is the key to becoming consciously aware of spirit. In the "Meditation" chapter in *A Search for God* it states: "Meditation is the safest and surest way to understand ourselves. It is the key to the door which is closed on the real world for most of us. Let us study and know ourselves. It is a command, an entreaty. Let us dare to seek, not blindly, but with faith, that we may find 'the noble self.' "

I believe that my other dreams and my encounter with the moon were manifested from my own spirit. I depend more on my spirit now, probably because it was my dearly beloved companion during Ray's illness, and I never wanted the conscious awareness of my spirit to leave me.

I have no doubt in my heart that the Holy Spirit came for Ray the night he died to guide him through his radiant passage. I believe that the Holy Spirit enters to help all the dying, but we were fortunate enough to have conscious awareness to witness the event. I will never forget any of it. As I mentioned earlier, Cayce in one reading says that the Holy Spirit *is* Christ Consciousness. I have found this to be true. I also feel that the Holy Spirit is the messenger and heralder of the Christ Consciousness.

I realized how all the alternative forms of therapy seemed to be presented to us at just the right moment as we moved along Ray's journey. Our society fosters a deep belief in traditional medicine, and that belief often helps with healing. But we found our experience with alternative therapies to be an important adjunct to Ray's treatment and were astonished at what meditation, Reiki, and TRT accomplished for him. To anyone in the same situation that Ray and I were in, I'd say, be open to new ideas in healing and don't limit the patient only to accepted medical treatments. Even though there are success cases with traditional medicine, and Ray couldn't be one of those, throughout our ordeal we were hard put to see how it assists the soul, soothes the spirit, or even calms the emotions. Most doctors today are not exposed to those aspects of the healing process. Medicine is surely necessary to heal the physical body, but the physical, mental, emotional, and spiritual parts of us are all entwined. Little else makes sense but a holistic approach to healing the whole person rather than merely targeting a diseased cell.

When you or the one you love learns to find the quiet within, move into the use of visualization, which will open the door further into the spiritual. Using a book like Dr. Siegel's as a guide, try making a tape. You'll be amazed at the help it can render.

There are many holistic healing centers appearing now all across the country. If you can't find one, go to a health food store or alternative book store. They usually have a wide variety of related literature and can put you in touch with people who can help you. When you approach illness holistically, you and your loved one will find that you have some amount of control in the sickness. I found that feeling my power had been taken from me was terribly frustrating and one of the most difficult things for me to get used to. I could actually play a part in Ray's illness, as could he, by sharing in alternative methods of therapy.

We didn't get involved to any great degree with diet nor had there been time to use the Cayce remedies, an element of his psychic readings for which he is famous. By the time Ray was diagnosed with the cancer, it was so advanced that I don't believe any great change in diet would have mattered. What did matter greatly to me was the fact that, throughout his life, Ray had neither the right attitude nor any knowledge of proper food and nutrition. Our bodies have to be nourished properly to function well in the physical. It's a parent's responsibility to learn about food values and make sure that their children eat properly. If you're not knowledgeable about how the content of food affects the body, pick up a book and gain some insight. There are many who claim that they have cured cancer through diet. I wouldn't dispute anything after what I have seen, but I suspect that there must be a lot of spiritual balancing along with the special diet.

If you are a caregiver for someone who is terminally ill, let the person express himself or herself on every subject. It isn't difficult for the dying to speak of death; often the person wants to talk, and intimately. Prepare yourself to allow the individual to do this. Don't deny him or her the opportunity to relate to you on the deepest levels possible. If you yourself can't face talking with the patient about death, then just sit and listen. You can help greatly by just listening. These individuals are going on a journey; they want to talk about it. Don't keep telling them that everything is going to be all right. When the time comes, you must face the reality just as they are doing.

If a patient's illness is terminal and there is no chance for physical healing, then the mental, emotional, and spiritual elements are doubly important. Try to help these people prepare for their journey ahead. More important, don't try to hold them here by telling them that you can't live without them. Remember that they must move along on their journey independently of you. There will be a point of no return for them beyond which they must continue on to their definite destination alone.

If you can release them, you will accomplish so much both for the one who is ill and for yourself. Give them permission to leave—you'll know when the time is right to do that. Pray for yourself and your loved one and ask that you can accept whatever is the most beneficial for all involved. Above all, never loose your faith or your hope. Cayce often said, " . . . never worry as long as you can pray. When you can't pray—you'd better begin to worry! For then you have something to worry about!" (3569-1)

In May of 1987, Gina graduated from college. It was terribly difficult for her without her father being there to smile and hug and congratulate her. She cried the whole day, but she and the rest of us managed to get through it.

Shortly afterward, in August of 1987, Cindy was accepted into medical school. How proud Ray would have been to see Cindy reach her longtime goal. But we knew that he was watching from some other place, and Cindy held on to that belief. She felt the gift that she had been given, of seeing her father's soul leave, would help her immensely when she would eventually have to relate to dying patients.

Betsy, our nurse, was drawn toward intensive care and started working in a large hospital in Philadelphia. She now deals solely with very ill and sometimes dying patients. I don't know if her father's illness affected her decision, but she finds her work extremely fulfilling. She told me recently about a patient who had died. Immediately after death, she went over and opened the window. I asked her why she had done that, and she told me that she really never thought about it. She said that a lot of the nurses do the same thing.

I remember the summer of 1987, when a great school of dolphins washed ashore, dead from the pollution in the ocean along the Eastern seaboard. Perhaps the dolphins were trying to tell us to clean up our waters before it was too late for all of us. I felt my connection with Ray and the dolphins again. Had that been an unconscious precognitive vision that Ray had when he told me to look for the dolphins? I would like to think that he had a hand in where they turned up and that the warning for all of us was to clean up our waters.

It was early summer before I felt recovered enough to venture out to look for work. But another difficult situation arose nearly at the same time. Ray's mother, Eva, who had been battling Parkinson's disease, was diagnosed with Alzheimer's as well, and could no longer take care of herself.

After a depleting four-month stretch, during which my daughters and I did what we could, we eventually had to put her into a home.

Gina and I both had precognitive dreams that foretold of her passing, and the intercession of spirit in our lives continued to astound me and fill me with awe. In Gina's dream, however, Grandma Jessie appeared, as she had done right before Ray passed on.

In the dream Gina found herself in the hospital with both of her grandmothers in the same room. Each was in her own bed, and Gina was sitting there visiting. She said that Grandma Jessie seemed very real to her. Then she heard Grandma Jessie say to Grandma Eva, "What are you waiting for? Why are you staying there?"

Gina was upset and couldn't imagine why Grandma Jessie was talking like this. Then Grandma Eva said, "But I'm trying to leave, and it's not easy. I don't know how."

Grandma Jessie said, "Just leave."

Grandma Eva said, "I'm trying to have a heart attack, but I just can't." Then they both laid back down on the beds. Gina was terrified beyond words.

Grandma Jessie then took Gina out of the hospital and into a cemetery. Gina knew it wasn't located nearby, but she knew it wasn't that far away either. She was then shown a grave with the name T.E. Kamish, the name of my father, on it. Grandma Jessie then took her to a different cemetery and told her that this was where Grandma Eva should be buried. Gina saw an open grave and what looked like a bridal bouquet on the ground next to it.

She woke up and was anxious when she told me about the dream. I thought about it and found it interesting and also correct in its content. By her description, I knew that the first cemetery to which my mother Jessie had taken Gina was in Brooklyn, where my father, T.E. Kamish, was buried. Gina had never been there before. Then Jessie took Gina farther, though not very far, to a different cemetery. This had to be in Fairlawn, in northern New Jersey, where Eva's family plot was, about a two-hour ride from Brooklyn. Gina was almost in tears when she told me about the dream, because she thought the bridal bouquet near the grave was somehow linked to her forthcoming marriage that June. However, Gina's fear of a death being connected to her marriage didn't touch me with truth. I knew that my mother, Jessie, was trying to tell us something important, but I couldn't figure it out. I told Gina that we would have to wait and see. I was concerned, though, as we each had a dream foretelling Eva's death.

It was only two days after Eva entered the home in early December, fourteen months following Ray's transition, that she passed on. We then found ourselves attending another funeral. The doctor suspected she had had a massive heart attack. We were all stunned and couldn't believe that she had left us so suddenly. We were sorely disappointed and upset that no one had been with her when she died. But then I realized that Eva probably would not have wanted us there, because we had been so positive with her. Her death was so sad. But going over what had transpired recently in her life, I sensed it was probably her wish because she knew she would not recover from Parkinson's and Alzheimer's. Further, she had recently lost her son.

Before her funeral, we experienced many serious family disagreements about where and how the funeral services should be conducted and where she should be buried. I knew Gina's dream held the answer, but I didn't quite understand it. Whatever it was, I knew it was important and that my mother, Jessie, was trying to tell us something. After the funeral services here in Pennsylvania for us and for Eva's close friends, we took her to her family burial plot in Fairlawn, New Jersey. I then saw that there were two separate graves aside from the large family plot. She had always told me about the family plot, but I couldn't remember her saying definitely that was where she wanted to be buried. Then I realized with sudden clarity that the bridal bouquet next to the open grave in Gina's dream was the clue! We were being told that Eva wanted to be buried with her husband in the dual grave next to, but not in, her large family plot. I was truly amazed at the descriptive content of Gina's dream.

The second Christmas after Ray's passing came shortly after the funeral, another sad holiday for us. It had been a little over a year since Ray was gone, and now we had lost Grandma Eva, too, only three weeks before. Betsy and I couldn't bring ourselves to get the ornaments down from the attic. It wasn't until Luke went up by himself and started to haul them down that we decided to try to get involved, even if it were just for the children.

The following May of 1988, Holly graduated from college. It had been extremely demanding for her, but she managed to complete her education while caring for the girls and working part-time.

In June of 1988, we all went to Banbridge, County Down, Northern Ireland, for Gina and Brian's wedding. Thirty-five of our friends and relatives traveled with us to attend the event. The wedding was magnificent; Gina's sisters were among her six bridesmaids, and Sarah was flower girl. Ray was there, too, though not in the physical. Even though my brother gave Gina away, her father stood there in attendance. We saw him in the eye of our memories, tall and strong and handsome as he used to be, smiling at all of us.

After the wedding, a group of us toured Scotland, then we returned home. It was heart-wrenching to leave Gina. We knew that she would be flying back and forth to visit, but I felt with her wedding that I was losing someone else.

In December of 1988, Betsy remarried her ex-husband, Jerry, and since then they have added three more children to their family: Maggie, Caty, and Zach. This gives me a total of seven grandchildren, whom I love and enjoy more every day. Betsy is still an R.N. in intensive care in Philadelphia.

In August of 1989, Holly entered law school in Delaware. Because she was by herself with the two children, I moved to Delaware with her during that chaotic first year of school. I had no trouble landing a year's work assignment immediately. I came back to Pennsylvania after that first year, and Holly transferred to California to try to reconcile with her husband and finish law school there. We all flew out to California in May of 1991 to attend her graduation. How happy and proud we were of her achievement! In the ensuing years, Ray had missed so much. We never again felt like a complete unit after he left us. But life moved on, and Holly's triumph was a masterpiece. We sensed Ray in attendance during her graduation, too, and again he was smiling down on us. I was able to finally let go of Ray that year.

Ray had loved the northern California beaches, so I brought his ashes with me. There was a beautiful beach that curved like a crescent moon along the coast, with huge stands of rock guarding the shoreline. I walked the beach one sunny morning and with a calmness in my heart scattered Ray's ashes into the outgoing tide. It didn't seem like a forever kind of goodby, though. I sat for awhile on the beach in peace and spoke inwardly with him. I felt very close to him and knew that we could be together again in some other time and place if that was our choice. Somehow I knew that maybe it wouldn't happen in the next lifetime or the one after that, but there was another journey for us that was still unfinished.

Holly's attempted reconciliation failed, but she felt that she had given it her all. I told her at the time that I was sure she had other things to accomplish in this lifetime. She now works for a fine law firm and is still living in California.

The following week, in June of 1991, Cindy graduated from medical school, finally reaching her goal that had been with her since she had been small. What an accomplishment my oldest daughter had achieved! We were so proud of her, and so sad that her father wasn't there to see it. But, again, we knew that he was aware of her triumph. Cindy is a surgical resident now in a local hospital and will be a caring and dedicated surgeon in a few years. It has been a long, long haul for her, but she loves her work, and there is nothing else that she would rather do.

My encounters with the guiding light of spirit didn't end there. Spirit constantly nudged me, and then at times would suddenly shove me. In October of 1991 I was in a movie theatre with Annmarie. It was about three minutes to eight and we were waiting for the show to start. Suddenly I heard powerful rumblings and had the sensation of my seat shaking. I looked around, and no one had noticed. The rumbling got much louder and the sense of shaking increased. I looked at Annmarie. She was sitting next to me quietly eating her popcorn.

"What is that?" I asked her. She said she hadn't heard anything.

The noise increased tremendously, and I said to her, "It sounds like an earthquake." The noise stopped within the next few minutes, so I figured it had to be something outside. I thought about that later and realized that I never seem to catch on immediately when an encounter occurs, but instead I try to apply logic to the situation. I arrived home from the movies about 11:00 p.m. The TV was on. Betsy was in the living room and told me that they had a terrible earthquake in northern California at 5:00 p.m. and that she couldn't reach Holly on the telephone. I thought about what I had heard at 8:00 p.m. and suddenly realized that that was 5:00 p.m. California time. We spent hours waiting for Holly to get through on the phone and prayed constantly. When she finally called, she was very frightened and told us what a terrible experience it had been for her and the kids. Evidently I had tuned in on her while it was happening. That increased our anticipation in looking forward to the day when she would move back to Pennsylvania.

I became tired of working for the temporary agency, even though it had been varied and interesting over the years. I needed benefits now. In July of 1992, I received my paralegal certificate and started a new job.

Gina returned to the states in July of 1992 to work on her master's in psychology. She is back and forth to Ireland now and will consider applying to the doctorate program in another year. She gained a great deal of insight during the time her father was ill, and it will add to her understanding and caring for her patients in the future.

Even though I have faced great trauma, I consider myself one of the fortunate souls, because I have been given custody in this lifetime of four loving, caring, and sensitive daughters. I am thankful that they chose me as their mother and entered into my life to bring me such love. I was also blessed because God was there for me during Ray's illness, opening the heavens and showering help in abundance through my spirit. I will tell you again, "Ask and you will receive."

It was also emotionally difficult reliving those desperate seven months as I wrote this book from my journal. I wondered at times if I would be able to get through the memories which became so intensely alive for me once again. Perhaps it gave me a sense of what actually happened through that time, because living through it for me was nothing more than helplessly being there. While writing, I realized even more how much being in touch with spirit helped me. During that year, I could get no sense of proportion or import of the overall picture. Writing my book, however, gave me the needed, extended contact with Ray, enabling me to put our journey into perspective, and create a tribute to him that may help many others.

The most important motivation for me to write this information down was knowing that Ray wanted to share his conscious encounters so that perhaps he could help others see into the greater universal context.

His spirit would tell you—open your hearts with meditation, journey with visualization, and don't be afraid to touch unknown places within your psyche. Heal your soul with the universal energy from TRT, Reiki, or a host of other energy-work therapies, such as Mari-EL, Therapeutic Touch, or polarity therapy. Touch your inner self with the magnificent colors of God's rainbow. Let His spirit into your heart. All of these ideas are soul-healing, which in turn can lead you to physical, mental, and emotional balancing. The universe and all its wonders are within your reach; all you have to do is acknowledge spirit and spirit will do the rest.

There was also a greater truth in what Ray discovered. The physical is fleeting; the spirit is constant and eternal. We are human and cannot understand another's mission from this earthly perspective. Never judge another; every entity faces self, and each has his or her own way of healing self. One way is not better than another. Have faith that spirit is always with you. Open your ears and eyes to receive it. Ray's spirit was eternal and invincible, and that was his lesson to us. The conscious merging of our spirits was his gift to me. Supporting his soul was my gift to him.

> "We parted, and not a word was spoken, but at one and the same moment had we understood our inexpressible thought . . . We have never met again. Perhaps centuries will elapse before we do meet again.
>
> "Much is to learn, and much to forget,
> "Through worlds I shall traverse not a few
>
> before we shall again find ourselves *in the same*

movement of the soul as on that evening: but we can well afford to wait."

Maurice Maeterlinck
(*The Invisible Goodness*;
from *The Treasure of the Humble*,
trans. by Alfred Sutro)

As with all of life's experiences, my journey with Ray changed me both inwardly and outwardly forever. As Josef told me, I "moved a great deal," and I'm sure he meant upward in awareness. But Ray was responsible for that, too. The world is a beautiful place, and we who are part of it are a part of the whole; but we are also the whole. I'm sure I have a greater love and empathy for others now. I understand with my whole being that each of us is on a journey, and I truly wish every one of us, as people on a journey, godspeed. The passage is hard, but the terminus holds magnificent rewards.

Sometimes I still miss Ray terribly, and my human emotional side wishes he were here with me to play out the rest of our years. But when I need help, I still speak to him. There are times when I sense him strongly and feel there is something near my shoulder. There are other times when I sense he is far, far away, doing wonderful things. Love endures and never ends. It's only the way in which it presents itself at the moment that matters. The void has softened into happy memories that I thought initially were lost, and the terrible difficulty of getting past the physical ravages of the illness is starting to fade. I can remember Ray now as he was before the sickness came. And I am grateful.

About the Author

Jeanette Fusco's interests and hobbies are varied and diverse. Through her ongoing studies in metaphysics, shamanism, dream interpretation, and the Edgar Cayce readings, she continues to seek helpful insights into the art of everyday living.

Her hobbies include painting, geneology, and astrology, along with designing and sewing children's clothes which she sold professionally in her own boutique some years ago. After living in various areas of the country and seeing most of the United States, she traveled extensively in Europe and would like to do more traveling after she retires.

Jeanette works as a paralegal and finds the field of law fascinating. She lives in the Philadelphia area with her Norwegian elkhound, Prince Orion of Norway, and her cat Fluffy. She spends time with her seven grandchildren and four daughters, who live in Pennsylvania, Northern Ireland, and California.

Jeanette is currently writing a children's mystery book.

What Is A.R.E.?

The Association for Research and Enlightenment, Inc. (A.R.E.®), is the international headquarters for the work of Edgar Cayce (1877-1945), who is considered the best-documented psychic of the twentieth century. Founded in 1931, the A.R.E. consists of a community of people from all walks of life and spiritual traditions, who have found meaningful and life-transformative insights from the readings of Edgar Cayce.

Although A.R.E. headquarters is located in Virginia Beach, Virginia—where visitors are always welcome—the A.R.E. community is a global network of individuals who offer conferences, educational activities, and fellowship around the world. People of every age are invited to participate in programs that focus on such topics as holistic health, dreams, reincarnation, ESP, the power of the mind, meditation, and personal spirituality.

In addition to study groups and various activities, the A.R.E. offers membership benefits and services, a bimonthly magazine, a newsletter, extracts from the Cayce readings, conferences, international tours, a massage school curriculum, an impressive volunteer network, a retreat-type camp for children and adults, and A.R.E. contacts around the world. A.R.E. also maintains an affiliation with Atlantic University, which offers a master's degree program in Transpersonal Studies.

For additional information about A.R.E. activities hosted near you, please contact:

A.R.E.
67th St. and Atlantic Ave.
P.O. Box 595
Virginia Beach, VA 23451-0595
(804) 428-3588

A.R.E. Press

A.R.E. Press is a publisher and distributor of books, audio-tapes, and videos that offer guidance for a more fulfilling life. Our products are based on, or are compatible with, the concepts in the psychic readings of Edgar Cayce.

We especially seek to create products which carry forward the inspirational story of individuals who have made practical application of the Cayce legacy.

For a free catalog, please write to A.R.E. Press at the address below or call toll free 1-800-723-1112. For any other information, please call 804-428-3588.

A.R.E. Press
Sixty-Eighth & Atlantic Avenue
P.O. Box 656
Virginia Beach, VA 23451-0656